KU-285-084

CANCER: Science and Society

A SERIES OF BOOKS IN BIOLOGY
Cedric I. Davern, EDITOR

CANCER:
Science
and
Society

John Cairns

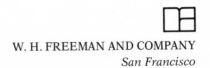

W. H. FREEMAN AND COMPANY
San Francisco

Cover illustration from *Kermesse at Hoboken* by Breughel.
Courtesy of the Courtauld Institute of Art, London.

Library of Congress Cataloging in Publication Data

Cairns, John.
    Cancer: science and society.

    (A Series of books in biology)
    Bibliography: p.
    Includes index.
    1. Cancer. I. Title. [DNLM: 1. Neoplasms—
Popular works. QZ201 C136c]
RC261.C252   616.9'94   78–16960
ISBN 0–7167–0098–0
ISBN 0–7167–0097–2 pbk.

Printed in the United States of America

9 8 7 6 5 4 3 2 1

CONTENTS

PREFACE

This book is a nontechnical account of the cancer problem and has been written with two quite different audiences in mind. The first is the general public—people who are interested in cancer because it is a disease that may affect them or their families. Not having a scientific background, some of these readers may find that the two chapters on experimental cancer research are abstruse and demand too great an effort; if they do, they should skip them and proceed to Chapter 9. The second audience consists of medical students and undergraduates in the biological sciences who are perhaps considering a career in cancer research; they may think that parts of the book are oversimplified, and for them references to more technical accounts are provided throughout the text.

My aim is to give an overall review of what is known about cancer—the nature of the disease, its causes, its importance in relation to other diseases and preoccupations of contemporary society, and the possibilities for its ultimate conquest. I would also like to tell the reader something about the state of the relevant sectors of biology, because it will surely be through science (rather than luck or some feat of alchemy) that cancer will finally be conquered. Therefore, in order to understand the prospects, people should have some idea of the present state of certain sciences.

The book is certainly not meant to be a kind of consumer's guide to cancer. Indeed, I have gone out of my way to avoid discussing the accepted treatments and probable outcome for each type of cancer, even though this has meant somewhat underplaying the advances of modern medicine and surgery. Also, rather than making any firm pronouncements on what are likely to be the most fruitful forms of cancer research, I have tried to show how the subject touches on many different disciplines ranging from chemistry and biology to economics and politics.

In fact, the book underwent two metamorphoses. At first I had intended to write a compendious review of the whole subject—the work I wished I myself could have read on first entering the field. As a displacement activity and relief from that seemingly unending task, I agreed to prepare a short article about cancer for *Scientific American*. And that eventually led me to revise my initial plan and undertake the much more reasonable exercise of writing a book for the general public.

Probably more than most authors, I have been helped by others. First and foremost of my advisers was Bruce Ponder whose interest, enthusiasm, and hard work got the final version moving again after it had been stalled for a long time in the section on experimental cancer research; without his aid the book might never have been finished. At several stages the various manuscripts were read and criticized by David Dressler, Brigid Hogan, and Richard Peto, and I am grateful to them for innumerable suggestions. For certain matters of fact, emphasis, or grammar I am indebted to Cedric Davern, Richard Doll, Linus Pauling, and Miranda Robertson. And for general comfort and advice, I am indebted to my wife and children.

The final text owes a great deal to Michele Liapes, of W. H. Freeman and Company, who has sifted through it indefatigably in search of ambiguities and obscurities. For the cover, we are very grateful to the Courtauld Institute of Art, London, for permission to reproduce the drawing *Kermesse at Hoboken* by Breughel. Last, I am pleased to acknowledge the support I have received, first from the American Cancer Society and then from the Imperial Cancer Research Fund, during the time I have been working on the book.

June, 1978   John Cairns

CANCER: Science and Society

INTRODUCTION 1

In the modern industrialized world, where famine and pestilence are things of the past, cancer has become the most feared of all diseases. It may not be the commonest cause of death, occurring much less frequently than heart disease, but it has the reputation of being usually a progressive fatal condition for which no treatment has been discovered. Further, the very nature of cancer makes it seem a particularly unnecessary form of death. By way of comparison, although the immediate cause of death in a heart attack is a local abnormality of the arteries supplying the heart, the underlying condition is a widespread defect affecting other parts of the body as well. So we tend to think of a heart attack as just one particular manifestation of the general process of aging, and a normal end to a long life; or, when it occurs in a man who is still middle-aged, as the price he has paid for overeating, lack of exercise, and a life of stress. But cancer is seen as something that originates in one localized region and then spreads so that the rest of the body, which would otherwise still be healthy, is gradually eaten away by the disease.

Each case of cancer originates as a defect in one of our cells that allows it to start multiplying and give rise to an ever increasing population of similarly unrestrained progeny cells. The first symptom produced by this population of multiplying cells depends on their location. If they arise in the skin, for example, they will produce a rapidly detected growth; in the lung they might cause a persistent cough or an unexplained attack of pneumonia; in the breast they may be detected simply as a lump (tumor). The patient consults a doctor, and a provisional diagnosis of cancer is made, perhaps on the basis of X-rays or a biopsy (the microscopic examination of a small sample excised from the tumor). In most instances, the best treatment is then to remove the tumor surgically. If the entire population of cells can be excised, this procedure will produce a complete cure. However, a common characteristic of such abnormal cells is that they acquire the ability to invade the surrounding tissues and spread by way of the blood and lymph systems to form secondary deposits *(metastases)* in distant sites. If this invasion has already occurred by the time of first diagnosis, excision of the primary tumor will not produce a cure, and other methods of treatment such as X-irradiation or chemotherapy will have to be used; unfortunately, these additional methods of treatment are not very effective for most forms of cancer.

The outcome depends, therefore, on whether the abnormal population of cells has extended beyond the original site, and the likelihood that there has been spread varies greatly according to the kind of cell affected. For example, most cancers of the skin do not readily undergo metastasis and for that reason, even though very common, they are not often lethal. At the other extreme, cancer of the lung is seldom detected before metastases have occurred.

The probable behavior of the different kinds of cancer and their response to the different forms of treatment have been determined over the years, and this knowledge is the basis for selecting the proper treatment for each case. The information is, however, totally empirical and has not been converted into any general theory of cancer.

For the outsider who tries to review the entire field, it is possible to see in the cancer problem a reflection of the problems of contemporary society. We are living in an age of transition. Once everything seemed within our reach; now we see limits whichever way we turn. We succeed in virtually abolishing mortality in the young, and a population explosion results. We then succeed in reducing the birth rate, but as the proportion of children in the population falls the proportion of old people starts to rise. We invent ever more effective offensive weapons with which to defend ourselves, and our safety from attack becomes more and more uncertain. We learn how we could easily prevent the most lethal of all cancers (lung cancer), and people continue to smoke. However, it looks as if cancer research is soon going to offer additional options, and before long society may be able to decide what exactly it wishes to do about each kind of cancer— whether to prevent it, spend vast sums of money treating it, or let it run its course. Some of these problems are described in the following chapters.

CANCER 2
and the CHANGING
PATTERN of MORTALITY

During the past 150 years, there has been a progressive elimination of infectious diseases as a major cause of death, and because most children now survive to reproductive age a sudden population explosion has ensued. In the United States, life expectancy has risen from roughly 30 years to 70. This has brought into prominence the diseases peculiar to old age, particularly cardiovascular disease and cancer.

During the past 150 years the Western world has virtually eliminated death due to infectious diseases. As a result, cancer and cardiovascular disease have replaced them as the major causes of mortality, and cancer has become the most publicized problem for applied biology. However, before describing what is known about the origins and nature of cancer, we should first consider how the general pattern of mortality in our society has been changing. We in the West are living through the final stages of a period of expansion and are about to experience a major change in the age distribution of our population. This is going to force us to revise our lifestyle and the way we look upon the different causes of death.

Past Changes in Age-Specific Mortality

For most of the time man has been on the earth, the total population increased very slowly.[1] Mortality was high, especially in infancy, meaning that each adult woman had to bear six children, on the average, in order to ensure that one daughter would survive to produce the next generation. Occasionally some innovation, like the invention of agriculture or the discovery of the principle of rotating crops, might suddenly raise the countryside's capacity for supporting people, and there would be a temporary increase in the birth rate or decrease in mortality; and then the population would stabilize at its new level. Occasionally, some catastrophic famine or pestilence would occur, and then, because fertility and mortality were so delicately balanced, many generations would have to elapse before the original numbers had been restored.

Minor differences undoubtedly existed between the death rates in different cultures, but basically the pattern of mortality did not undergo any major change until the mid-19th century. What happened then is still somewhat unclear. Various agricultural reforms had spread through Europe in the 17th and 18th centuries, and these had raised the productivity of the land and had produced a minor increase in population. But then came the Industrial Revolution, and by the middle of the 19th century a population explosion was well under way in all Western nations. It was not due to any increase in fertility; indeed, the birth rate in most industrialized nations was steadily drifting downwards throughout the 19th century. Instead, what had occurred was a sudden drop in mortality which allowed a greater proportion of children to survive and reproduce.

The causes for this decline in mortality are not well understood, because it began before the advent, in the 20th century, of what we would call medical science.[2] For example, in 1837 England became one of the first countries to start keeping an annual register of births and deaths, and these records plainly show that much of the huge reduction in death rate since then had already taken place by 1900 (Figure 2-1).[3]

The record is, of course, more reliable in the matter of the number of deaths than the exact causes of deaths, but the early statisticians were probably correct in ascribing nearly all the deaths in youth and middle age to infectious diseases such as tuberculosis, dysentery, typhoid, and diphtheria. There was no

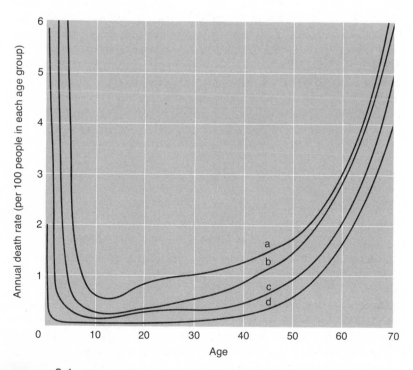

FIGURE 2-1   The relation between age and death rate (percent dying each year) in England for the periods (a) 1841–1850, (b) 1901–1910, (c) 1931–1940, and (d) 1961–1970.

specific treatment for any of these diseases in the 19th century, and so the mortality from them could have been reduced only by general measures of hygiene and public health—i.e., improvement in nutrition, housing, water supplies, and sewage. Later, in the 20th century, the eradication of infectious diseases in industrialized countries was effectively completed by vaccines and antibiotics. It is significant, however, that what is often thought of as one of the accomplishments of sophisticated medical science was, in large part, the product of some fairly simple improvements in public health. In the end, history may well repeat itself and the same prove to be true for cancer.

We can look at these statistics from two points of view: individual and national. Figure 2-1 shows how annual mortality for various age groups changed in one country (England) between 1850 and 1970—i.e., it shows the shift in the average person's probability of dying, in relation to age. But we can also look at the numbers for any country as a whole, and then compare how the deaths were divided among the different age groups at different periods of history. As Figure 2-2 shows, there was extraordinarily little change in the distribution of deaths between 10,000 B.C. and 1850 A.D. The really big change has come in the last 100 years of man's history. Apart from infant mortality, deaths used to be spread fairly evenly over all age groups. By 1972, however, more than 80% of all deaths were in people past the age of 60. In other words, death has now become largely relegated to old age.

The Present-Day Causes of Mortality

In Western societies, approximately 1% of the population dies every year; (the value would be 1.25% for a nonexpanding society in which each person lived for exactly 80 years, but for the time being the percentage is lower because, with a few exceptions like East Berlin, the population of every country has a disproportionately large number of children). For example, in the United States with its population of slightly over 200 million, about 1,900,000 people die each year. Roughly half these deaths are due to arterial disease, which can be directly fatal when it affects the arteries supplying the heart muscle and the brain, causing coronary thrombosis (heart attack) and cerebral vascular disease (stroke). The next major cause of death is cancer; it and the arterial diseases account for two-thirds of all deaths. The remaining

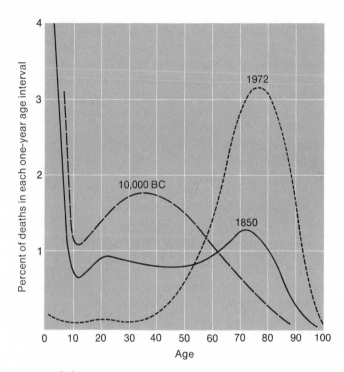

FIGURE 2-2   The age distribution of all the deaths (excluding infant mortality) that occurred in England in 1850 and 1972. These are compared to the distribution of the ages of the skeletons in two Mesolithic burial sites dating from about 10,000 B.C. [After *The Registrar General's Statistical Review of England and Wales for the Year 1972*, Part I, "Tables, Medical," H. M. Stationery Office (1974); D. E. Dumond, *Science* **187**, 713–721 (1975).]

one-third is due to respiratory diseases, accidents, congenital disorders, violence, and other causes. But the infectious diseases, which once ruled supreme, now cause only about 1% of all the deaths (Table 2-1).

Now, it could reasonably be argued that a table like this is almost useless without some further qualification. About 1% of the population in the United States is going to die every year, and so the table will list about two million deaths, come what may. Rather than the raw numbers, what we need is some measure of the untimeliness of the deaths so that we can see which causes of death represent the greatest loss. For the fact is that we are *not* diminished equally by every death; a twenty-year-old dying of leukemia is surely a greater loss than a ninety-year-old dying of

TABLE 2-1	Mortality in the U.S. in 1968	
Cause	Number of deaths	Percent of total
Vascular diseases		
Heart disease	674,747	35
Cerebral vascular diseases	211,390	11
Other	154,155	8
Total	1,040,292	54
All forms of cancer	318,547	17
Accidents and violence		
Automobile accidents	54,862	3
Other accidents	64,317	3
Suicide	21,372	1
Homicide	14,686	1
Total	155,237	8
Respiratory diseases	123,440	6
Infant mortality	43,840	2
Congenital abnormalities	16,793	1
Infectious diseases	17,776	1
Total	1,715,925	89
All causes	1,930,082	100

SOURCE U.S. Department of Health, Education, and Welfare. *Vital Statistics of the United States.* Volume II. *Mortality.* Washington, D.C.: U.S. Government Printing Office, 1972

cancer of the prostate. Obviously there is no totally satisfactory way of quantifying an abstract quality such as "loss," because much depends on what we consider a reasonable lifespan. I have chosen, for purposes of this discussion, one of the simpler methods, namely to calculate the loss of *working lifespan*—the 45 years between 20 and 65; deaths occurring at any time before the age of 20 count as the loss of 45 years, deaths after 65 do not count at all, and each death between 20 and 65 counts according to the number of years before 65 that it occurred. It should be recognized that what is being calculated here is the degree to which the different causes of death deprive people of their right to a reasonable lifespan, not the extent to which these causes erode the nation's work force.

Table 2-2 shows the major causes of death in the United States, arranged in their order of importance as causes of loss of working lifespan (in Chapter 3, the same procedure will be applied to the individual varieties of cancer). The main effect of perceiving mortality this way is that accidents move to the top of the table as the major cause. We see that the elimination of automobile accidents

Cause	Work years lost*	Percent of total
TABLE 2-2 Loss of working lifespan in the U.S. in 1968 from various causes		
Accidents and violence		
Automobile accidents	1,533,102	11
Other accidents	1,262,415	9
Homicide	397,668	3
Suicide	389,733	3
Total	3,582,918	26
Vascular diseases		
Heart disease	1,610,142	12
Cerebral vascular diseases	431,973	3
Other	578,801	4
Total	2,620,916	19
Infant mortality	1,970,489	14
Cancer	1,744,189	13
Respiratory diseases	968,064	7
Congenital diseases	674,465	5
Infectious diseases	291,185	2
Total	11,852,226	86
All causes	13,687,716	100

*Working life is considered to extend for 45 years, from age 20 to age 65. Deaths occurring before the age of 20 each contribute 45 lost years to the total, and those occurring between 20 and 65 contribute appropriately fewer, and deaths after 65 do not count.

would save about as much working lifespan as the cure of cancer. In fact, it may turn out to be easier to design a safer automobile that offers better protection for the driver and passengers than to prevent deaths caused by the main varieties of cancer.

Tables such as 2-1 and 2-2 are a convenient way of listing a large number of different causes of death. But if we are considering just the differences in the *patterns* of death due to a few selected causes, these are most clearly shown in a graph, such as Figure 2-3.

Future Changes in Population and Mortality

Having learned how to eradicate most mortality under the age of 40, the West has exported this technology to many other countries and thereby created a worldwide population explosion. The increase in growth rate is, of course, bound to be transient, for eventually something will become limiting in each country and

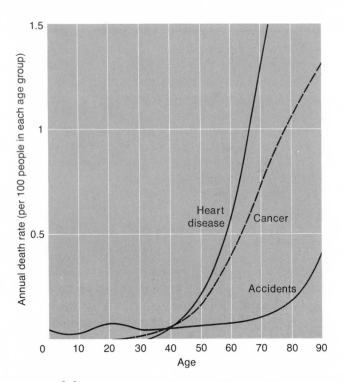

FIGURE 2-3   The relation in the United States, 1968, between age and the percent of people who die each year from ischemic heart disease, cancer, or an accident. [After U.S. Department of Health, Education, and Welfare. *Vital Statistics of the United States.* Volume II. *Mortality.* U.S. Government Printing Office, 1968.]

the growth will level off. In principle, stabilization could be brought about either by a reduction in birth rate or by a return of high mortality before the age of reproduction. It is doubtful whether many countries would willingly accept an increase in mortality. So we may reasonably assume that sooner or later a worldwide reduction in birth rate will occur.

In many Western countries this has already occurred and each breeding female is now producing, on average, approximately two children, the number now required to ensure replacement of the breeding population. The change is very recent, however, and most of these countries, like the United States, have an excess of children dating from the last few years of population growth, who are about to start breeding. So a generation must elapse before the total population stops increasing.

Irrespective of the final size of the stabilized population, we can easily calculate what its final age distribution will be if the mortality of each age group remains exactly at its present level; at the same time we can also work out what the age distribution would be if there were no deaths from cancer. As Figure 2-4 shows, we are going to have to face a tremendous change in the age distribution of the population, once zero growth has been established. As the two stabilization curves demonstrate, this shift in age distribution will dwarf the potential effects of cancer research because the total eradication of all forms of cancer would raise life expectancy by only two years. (This may seem a marginal gain for a lot of effort, but it is important to realize what these two years represent—namely that the one person in six who dies of cancer would otherwise have lived, on the average, for another twelve years before dying from some other cause; for those people, and their relatives, cancer research will have been worthwhile).

The main implication of the change is economic. At present, 10% of the population is over the age of 65. This will rise to 16% once zero growth has been attained (or to 18% if by that time we

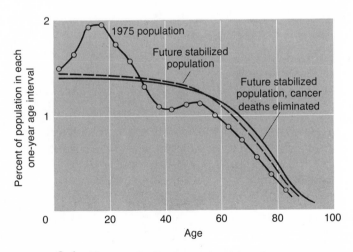

FIGURE 2-4 The age distribution of the United States population for 1975, compared with the distributions projected for populations that have stabilized, if age-specific mortality has been kept at its present level (broken line) or if all mortality due to cancer has been eliminated (solid line).

have conquered cancer). Somehow society must be organized to handle these large numbers of old people, without subjecting them to unacceptable hardship.[4] No country has ever had to face this problem before, because zero growth and low mortality have never occurred at the same time. Its solution seems to be at least as important a goal as the conquest of cancer.

The ORIGIN 3
and VARIETIES
of CANCER

Cancers can arise in any organ of the body, but some sites are more frequently affected than others. Each cancer is descended from a single cell that at some stage became free from its normal territorial restraints and so was able to form a family of cells that could multiply without limit.

The human body contains roughly ten million million (10^{13}) cells,[1] that are subdivided into groups and classes to form the various tissues and organs and are programmed to carry out various appropriate functions. Some of the cells (e.g., nerve cells) are apparently incapable of further division once they have been formed during development of the embryo or in infancy. Others, such as liver cells, seldom divide during our adult life but are capable of rapid multiplication on demand—for example after partial destruction of the liver. Still others, like those that form skin and the circulating cells of the blood, are continually having to divide throughout life in order to replace the cells that are lost or destroyed.[2] The multiplication patterns of certain cell types are shown in Figure 3-1. The whole edifice is, of course, the product of the division of a single cell and its descendants. From start to finish, from the fertilized egg to death in old age, a human being is the product of about 10^{16} cell divisions.

Obviously, in tissues where the cells multiply continuously, the total number of cells will remain constant only if cell death and emigration are exactly matched by cell production. Thus every part of the program of cell division, both in the embryo and in the adult, must be under very strict control. The possible nature of these controls will be discussed later. For the moment it is sufficient to see that a system like this will be open to Darwinian Selection. We may therefore expect occasional cell variants to develop that show increased "fitness" (i.e., that can multiply faster than normal or can displace their neighbors whenever space is limited). And in fact that is exactly what we observe. Families of cells can emerge that increase in number at the expense of their neighbors. When they multiply without some of the usual restraints (i.e., when they divide more frequently or are subject to less loss) but nevertheless keep within their normal territory and do not invade the surrounding tissues, they form *benign tumors;* examples range from the small cutaneous mole (of which most of us have a dozen or so) to the fairly common uterine "fibroid" which if not removed can sometimes become very large. If the abnormal cells have acquired the ability to spread to alien sites such as into neighboring tissues or to distant regions by way of the circulation, they are called *malignant tumors* or *cancers.* The distinction between these two classes of uncontrolled growth is all-important. It is the ability of a cancer to spread to multiple and distant sites that allows it to pass beyond the reach of local surgery.

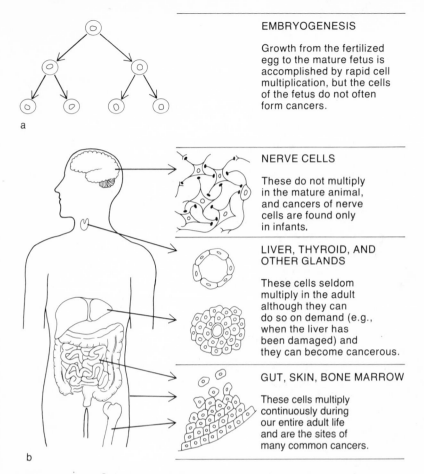

EMBRYOGENESIS

Growth from the fertilized egg to the mature fetus is accomplished by rapid cell multiplication, but the cells of the fetus do not often form cancers.

NERVE CELLS

These do not multiply in the mature animal, and cancers of nerve cells are found only in infants.

LIVER, THYROID, AND OTHER GLANDS

These cells seldom multiply in the adult although they can do so on demand (e.g., when the liver has been damaged) and they can become cancerous.

GUT, SKIN, BONE MARROW

These cells multiply continuously during our entire adult life and are the sites of many common cancers.

FIGURE 3-1   The multiplication of cells (a) in embroyogensis and (b) in different tissues of the body.

The Single-Cell Origin of Tumors

Before we go further into the classification of cancers and a description of their behavior, it is instructive to examine more closely the difference between the formation of a normal collection of apparently identical cells, like those of the liver, and the formation of a cancer. In recent years, several methods have been found for studying the lineage, or family tree, of cells during the formation and development of the embryo (embryogenesis). The simplest is to make use of an oddity of nature. It is important enough to describe in some detail because the concept of lineage is central to all our ideas about cancer.[3]

The sex of animals is usually determined by a particular pair of chromosomes. For example, in mammals these are the X chromosome and the Y chromosome; females are XX, having inherited an X from each parent; males are XY, having inherited one of their mother's X chromosomes and their father's Y chromosome. Now, unlike the other chromosomes, each of which is a member of an equally sized pair (one paternal in origin, one maternal) the Y chromosome is much smaller than the X. Therefore most of the X chromosome has no corresponding part in the Y and so, in males, has to operate alone. To maintain the same balance in females, which have two X chromosomes, one of the two is arranged not to function but is condensed into a tight package and set to one side in the nucleus. Now, the choice of which of a female's two X chromosomes should be inactivated in this way occurs irreversibly, early in embryogenesis, when there are perhaps only about 20 embryo cells present;[4] further, the choice made by each cell is apparently random and is irreversible (meaning that this choice is passed on to all of a cell's descendants). Thus every female is made up of a mixture of two kinds of cell—cells descended from those of the 20 that chose to inactivate the paternally derived X (X_p), and cells descended from the rest of the 20 that inactivated the maternal X (X_m). The behavior of the X chromosomes therefore makes each female into a *mosaic,* and this mosaicism can be demonstrated whenever the two X chromosomes differ in some distinguishable gene (Figure 3-2).

FIGURE 3-2   (a) Female mosaicism arising from X-chromosome inactivation. A female child contains two X chromosomes. This child is the result of the fusion of an egg, which bears one of her mother's two X chromosomes, with a sperm bearing her father's X chromosome; (a male child contains an X and a Y chromosome and results from the fusion of the X-bearing egg with a sperm bearing his father's Y chromosome). Early in the development of the female embryo, when the fertilized egg has multiplied to give probably about 20 fetal cells (the precise moment is not known exactly), the process of X-inactivation occurs. Each cell selects one of its two X chromosomes for inactivation: the choice is apparently made at random. As a result some of the cells are left with an active paternal X chromosome (X_p) and the others with an active maternal chromosome (X_m). Because the choice is never reversed, each female is therefore a *mosaic* of two kinds of cell. This mosaicism can be demonstrated whenever there happens to be some abnormality (i.e., mutation) of one of the two X chromosomes that leads to the presence of some detectably abnormal gene-product in all the cells in which the abnormal X is active. (b) Demonstration of the female mosaicism in certain adult tissues.

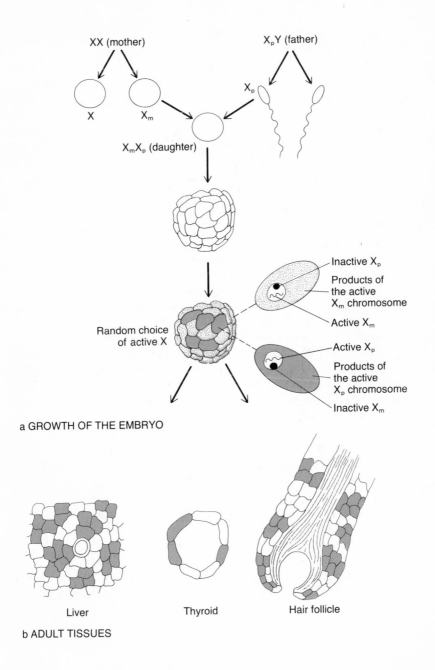

XX (mother)

X_pY (father)

X_p

X

X_m

X_mX_p (daughter)

Inactive X_p

Products of
the active
X_m chromosome

Active X_m

Random choice
of active X

Active X_p

Products of
the active
X_p chromosome

Inactive X_m

a GROWTH OF THE EMBRYO

Liver   Thyroid   Hair follicle

b ADULT TISSUES

The X chromosome marker most suitable for studies of human mosaicism is the gene for the enzyme glucose-6-phosphate-dehydrogenase (G6PD), which is involved in the breakdown of glucose in the cell. It so happens that certain variants of this enzyme confer some resistance to malaria and so are rather common in populations that are (or used to be) exposed to malaria. Thus quite a high proportion of black women are demonstrably mosaic for G6PD.

In such women it has been observed that the individual organs (e.g., liver), and even quite small collections of cells (e.g., the cells of individual hair follicles)[5] are almost invariably mosaic and therefore must have been descended from more than one of the 20 or so cells that were present at the time of X inactivation. Thus we see here the important principle that during embryogenesis each organ and tissue is not created from the descendants of a particular single cell. Instead, each organ is made up from the descendants of several different families of cells. Indeed, this would seem to be a rather reliable way of building the different parts of the body because there is no absolute need for any one particular cell to be in exactly the right place at the right time.

It turns out that tumors in such women are unlike the surrounding normal tissues in that they are found almost invariably to contain only one type of G6PD.[6] This is true whether the tumors are benign or malignant, implying that each tumor has arisen from a single cell.

Occasionally the same conclusion can be reached more directly. Certain cancers (e.g., some varieties of leukemia)[7] are associated with some particular visible chromosomal abnormality due, usually, to a piece of one chromosome having switched over to another (see p. 82). In these instances, one can observe that all the cancerous cells in the patient show exactly the same abnormality and so presumably are descended from a single cell that developed the abnormality and, perhaps because of that, gained the ability to multiply uncontrollably.

Thus the growth of a cancer is not like an epidemic spreading among normal cells but is the growth of a single family of abnormal cells (see Figure 3-3).

Classification of Cancer by Site

Most of the malignant invasive cancers of man belong to one of three groups. First and foremost come the *carcinomas*, which originate in the sheets of cells, or "epithelia," covering our surface

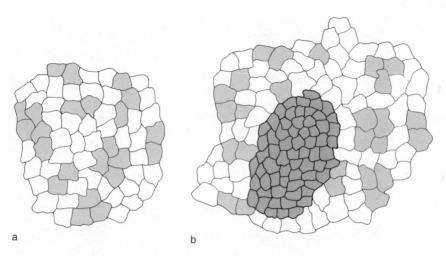

a   b

FIGURE 3-3   Benign tumors and malignant tumors (cancers) are expanding
families of cells derived from a single parent cell. Unlike normal tissues which
are mosaic—shown in (a) as a mixture of small families of white and shaded
cells—each cancer is a single family, as shown in (b).

(e.g., skin, respiratory tract, gut) and lining the various glands of
the body (e.g., breast, pancreas, thyroid). Next are the *sarcomas*,
which develop in the various supporting tissues of the body (such
as bone cells, blood vessels, fibrous tissue cells, muscle). Last is a
heterogeneous group of cancers originating in the cells that produce the circulating white cells of the blood (leukocytes) and the
immune system (i.e., the various kinds of lymphocyte); the classification of this third group is complicated and includes such
conditions as lymphosarcoma and Hodgkin's disease (which affect the lymph glands) and the various forms of leukemia (which
literally means an excess of white cells in the blood). The
terminology—like much that has developed in medicine—has
been built up gradually throughout the years, with little thought
given to creating a completely logical system. It is not an easy
language to learn, especially when it comes to the names of the
different types of cell that can form a cancer. As much as possible
the jargon of the pathologist will be avoided in this book, even at
the cost of an occasional circumlocution.

So much for the classification of cancers, according to cell type,
into the carcinomas of epithelial cells, the sarcomas of supporting
tissues, and the group that includes the leukemias. In fact, of
these three classes the carcinomas are numerically the most important. As Table 3-1 shows, more than 90% of human cancers

TABLE 3-1 Incidence of cancer in different classes of cell	
Class of cell	Percent of total*
Cancers of external epithelia, which are in immediate contact with the external environment (e.g., skin, large intestine, lung, stomach, cervix)	56
Cancers of internal epithelia (e.g., breast prostate, ovary, bladder, pancreas)	36
Cancers of the supporting tissues and blood-forming organs (the sarcomas and leukemias)	8

SOURCE   J. Clemmesen. "Statistical studies in malignant neoplasms." Acta Path. Microbiolo. Scand. Suppl. **174** (1964), **209** (1969), **247** (1974). The data in these three reports summarize the experience of the 4.5 million inhabitants of Denmark over 25 years. They were chosen because, unlike most national registries, the Danish Cancer Registry reports separately for each site the number of cancers that arose in the epithelial cells and the number of sarcomas arising in the supporting cells.

arise in epithelial cells (i.e., are carcinomas). Most of them originate in our surface epithelia which are in direct contact with the outside world, suggesting perhaps that the commonest causes of cancer may be agents that cannot penetrate very far. Less than 10% of the cancers of man arise in the supporting tissues of the body or the circulating cells (i.e., are sarcomas or leukemias). It is worth noting at this point that the distribution of cancers in animals is rather different from that shown here; for most of the animal species we know about, the leukemias and sarcomas are not nearly as rare.[8]

The further classification of cancers into different groups is according to the organ involved, or the type of cell involved when we are dealing with the nonlocalized cancers such as the leukemias. This is not a sterile academic exercise as we shall see when we come to consider the epidemiology of cancer, because it is quite clear that the different cancers have different causes.

In all, about 200 distinct varieties of cancer are recognized.[9] Fortunately, most of these are very rare, and we can encompass the majority of cancer mortality with a much smaller list. Table 3-2 lists the main varieties of cancer, according to the number of deaths each of them causes in the U.S. each year. Almost half of all the deaths are due to cancer of the lung, large intestine, and breast.

In the preceding chapter the various causes of death were listed—not only according to the actual number of deaths due to

TABLE 3-2   Mortality in the U.S.
in 1968 from the various cancers

Cancer site	Deaths	Percent of total
Lung	59,356*	19
Large intestine	44,431	14
Breast	29,075	9
Lymphomas	17,774	6
Pancreas	17,374	5
Stomach	16,900	5
Prostate	16,843	5
Leukemia	14,372	5
Ovary	9,488	3
Bladder	8,489	3
Brain	7,507	2
Cervix	7,106	2
Total	232,121	78
All cancers	318,495	100

SOURCE U.S. Department of Health, Education, and Welfare. *Vital Statistics of the United States.* Volume II. *Mortality.* Washington, D.C.: U.S. Government Printing Office, 1968.

*By 1976, deaths from lung cancer had risen to about 85,000 (i.e., to almost 25% of the total). [See American Cancer Society, "Cancer Incidence, 1976," *Ca-A Cancer Journal for Clinicians,* January/February (1976).]

each, but also the loss of working lifespan that they caused, on the grounds that we lose more from death of the young than from death of the old. Table 3-3 shows the same calculation made for some of the commoner kinds of cancer. Cancer of the lung (due almost entirely to cigarette smoking) still remains far ahead of the others; in fact, it is the only variety of cancer to cause more loss of lifespan than either homicide or suicide (see Table 2-2). The main difference between Tables 3-3 and 3-2 is that the leukemias and various cancers of the brain have moved up in importance because they occur not infrequently in children. Incidentally, this way of calculating the importance of various causes of death allows another comparison to be made. If we consider time spent in prison as in effect a loss of lifespan, then it is interesting to note that for men the total annual loss of lifespan in the United States due to imprisonment is about the same as that due to leukemia (for a variety of reasons fewer women go to prison, and so for them leukemia is much the greater hazard). It could be instructive for someone to compare the costs of research into possible ways of preventing imprisonment and leukemia, or

TABLE 3-3   Loss of working lifespan in the U.S. in 1968 from the various cancers

Cancer site	Work years lost	Percent of total
Lung	286,711*	16
Breast	208,328	12
Leukemia	175,973	10
Lymphoma	149,616	9
Large intestine	141,054	8
Brain	117,413	7
Cervix	67,690	4
Ovary	65,125	4
Pancreas	58,008	3
Stomach	51,420	3
Total	1,321,338	76
All cancers	1,744,189	100

SOURCE   J. L. Murray and L. M. Axtell. "Impact of cancer: years of life lost due to cancer mortality." *J. Natn. Cancer Inst.* **52**, 3–7 (1974).

*By 1976, loss of work years due to lung cancer had risen to about 400,000.

the costs of keeping people in prison and of treating cases of leukemia.

Classification by Cell Behavior

This chapter has thus far been concerned with the origin of cancers from single cells and the frequency of cancer in different sites, i.e., the classification according to gross anatomy. We must now examine briefly the way cancer cells multiply and spread, i.e., the classification according to their microscopic anatomy. As Table 3-1 showed, cancer in man is predominately a disease of epithelia. The anatomy and organization of a typical epithelium is well illustrated by the skin.[10] (See Figure 3-4.)

The epithelium of the skin is called the epidermis; it forms a sheet, usually five to 10 cells deep, overlying a loose-knit layer of supporting cells, the dermis. The epidermis continually replaces itself by the division of the cells in its deepest, or basal, layer next to the dermis.[11] As a result of this constant cell division, cells are continuously squeezed out of the basal layer into more superficial layers. There they begin to differentiate according to an established program: they flatten, begin to synthesize the insoluble protein keratin, and dissolve their nucleus. Finally they fuse into

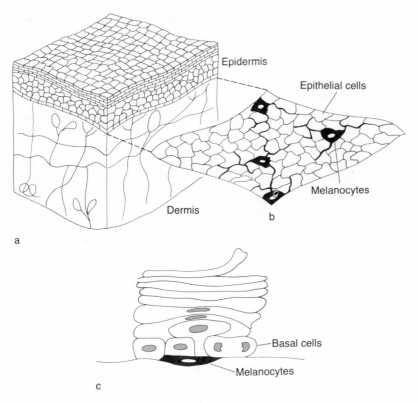

Epidermis

Epithelial cells

Melanocytes

Dermis

b

a

Basal cells

Melanocytes

c

FIGURE 3-4   (a) The division of skin into dermis (containing blood vessels, nerves, sweat glands) and epidermis.

(b) The plane view of the basal cells of the epidermis showing the arrangement of the interspersed melanocytes.

(c) An enlarged diagram of the epidermis showing the basement membrane between it and the underlying dermis, the dividing cells of the basal layer, and the more superficial cells that are losing their nuclei and differentiating to form flakes of keratin.

the keratin flakes called *squames,* which are eventually shed from the surface.[12] The result of this program of development is that we are separated from our immediate environment by a fairly impenetrable layer of insoluble keratin that is being continuously shed and replaced by the underlying "squamous" epithelium. (The behavior of the differentiating squamous epithelial cells of the skin is an instance of programmed cell death; probably the most familiar example is the death and release of leaves and fruit each autumn—processes that are plainly the result of an active program because they do not occur so quickly in trees that have died during the summer.)

In addition to epithelial cells, the epidermis also contains scattered pigment cells, or *melanocytes*, which synthesize granules containing the dark brown pigment melanin and donate these to the maturing epithelial cells. In this way the deeper layers of the skin, including the multiplying basal cells, are protected from ultraviolet light.

From the behavior of the epidermal cells we can deduce that they must be subject to several distinct forms of control. First, the fact that the only cells that divide are those in contact with the underlying dermis suggests that some short-range signals pass between the dermis and the basal cells; in the absence of these signals an epidermal cell stops multiplying and starts differentiating. Second, in order to prevent the multiplying basal cells from invading the dermis some mechanism must establish and enforce the boundary between the two layers. Third, some system of lateral signals must determine the even spacing of the melanocytes so that there are no gaps in our protection against ultraviolet light, and similar longer-range signals must regulate the spacing of epidermal structures such as hair follicles and sweat glands.

In addition to local regulation of growth, various overriding systems of control can be perceived in the behavior of the cells. Although surface characteristics such as fingerprints are expressed by the epidermis, they are determined by the dermis:[13] if epidermal tissue is removed from the thigh, for example, and grafted onto the palm, it will thicken and take on the pattern of lines characteristic of the palm. If an area of skin is subjected to increased wear, the program of differentiation is somehow modified to increase the depth of the epidermis and thicken the keratin layer, forming a callus. If an area is denuded of epithelium, it is recolonized by an increase in the rate of cell division in the surrounding epidermis. If exposure to sunlight is increased, the rate of pigment production is greatly accelerated. Finally, if a piece of skin becomes implanted into subcutaneous tissues (as can easily happen in an accident or as a result of a hypodermic injection), the skin is somehow programmed to die rather than multiply in an alien site.[14]

The means by which these controls are effected is not known. For example, the communication that is obviously occurring between epithelial cells and underlying dermis could be in the form of a concentration gradient (i.e., a difference in concentration between one layer and the adjacent one) of a freely diffusible substance secreted by some cells and detected by others (like the signaling system that is thought to control head regeneration in the simple freshwater animal called Hydra); this means that all the surface cells acquire a sense of direction and therefore "know" which way they are to move when they start on their program of development. Or the communication could require the kind of direct contact between the cells that is now thought to occur when signals pass between groups of cells at certain stages in embryonic development. Different examples of communication between cells are shown in Figure 3-5.[15] Whatever the mechanism, communication could be interrupted if there was a defect either in the signaler or in the recipient. Because there seem to be many signaling systems operating on skin epithelium, there should be many distinct varieties of uncontrolled growth—some that might lead to invasion and metastasis (i.e., be cancerous) and some that might not. And that is exactly what has been found.

For example, consider two well known noncancerous abnormalities of growth control of the skin, namely *psoriasis* and the common *wart*. In psoriasis the layer of multiplying basal cells extends about 10 cells deep,[16] and this seems to be due to some error of communication with the underlying dermis because psoriatic patches are reported never to extend over scar tissue.[17] The common wart, which is due to infection by a virus, shows a great thickening of all layers of the epithelium as if the progress of differentiation has been drastically slowed so that more cells are caught at each level of differentiation; but the overall arrangement of the epithelial cells remains precisely ordered and the boundary with the dermis is unchanged.

There are two common cancers of skin epithelium and one less common cancer originating in skin melanocytes; all three are usually induced by sunlight.[18] The *basal cell carcinoma*, as its name implies, apparently consists of cells derived from the basal layer of epithelium that seem to have escaped the control of the system that normally preserves the boundary between the dermis and the epidermis. Its cells invade the dermis and the underlying tissues, forming an irregular erosive ulcer (hence its other name of "rodent ulcer");[19] but despite its great capacity for local invasion, this form of skin cancer virtually never spreads to distant

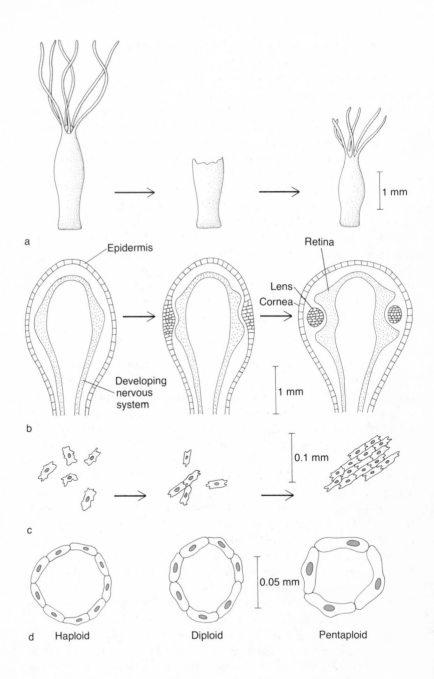

a

b

Epidermis

Retina

Lens
Cornea

Developing
nervous
system

1 mm

1 mm

c

0.1 mm

d   Haploid   Diploid   Pentaploid

0.05 mm

sites by way of the blood stream or lymphatics, suggesting perhaps that its cells still require signals from skin dermis in order to multiply. The other common epithelial cancer of skin, the *squamous carcinoma*, is similarly made up of disordered groups of cells but these undergo almost normal differentiation into squames of keratin; it tends not to be as locally invasive as the basal cell carcinoma but it can occasionally give rise to distant deposits (*metastases*). These four types of abnormal skin growth are shown in Figure 3-6.

The cancer that arises in melanocytes is called *malignant melanoma*. It is quite rare, and this is fortunate because it has a notorious tendency to undergo rapid and extensive metastasis. This property may perhaps be related to the developmental history of the ancestor of the melanocyte (the *melanoblast*), which arises in the embryonic central nervous system and migrates out from there to colonize the rest of the body including the skin; thus melanoblasts are born to be invaders, programmed from the start to move apart from each other, and indeed they will show this property when brought together in a confined space *in vitro*.[20]

FIGURE 3-5   Examples of communication between cells.

(a) Regeneration in Hydra. In this small freshwater animal, the foot and the head and tentacles signal their presence by producing freely diffusible substances that form concentration gradients up and down the body. When the head is cut off, the gradients are altered and the cells in the stump become programmed to multiply and regenerate a new head.

(b) Development of the vertebrate eye from the embryonic nervous system and the overlying surface cells (ectoderm). The developing brain forms two outgrowths (the optic vesicles, or future retinas), which proceed to trigger proliferation and infolding of the ectoderm to make the lens and cornea. This interaction between nervous system and ectoderm is probably due to signals that are transferred by direct cell contact.

(c) The first steps in development of the fruiting body of the slime mold. When food runs out, these free-living amoebas summon each other together by emitting short pulses of a diffusible signal (which is known to be cAMP—cyclic adenosine monophosphate—in some species of amoeba). This is therefore a particularly clear example of cell interactions that produce order out of chaos; superficially, at least, it is potentially a model of carcinogenesis in reverse.

(d) Even such simple things as the width of the tubules in the kidney are determined by the interaction of the tubule cells with the surrounding supporting tissue. Thus, even though the size of the cells is greatly altered in animals that have fewer or extra sets of chromosomes, the diameter of the tubules remains unchanged. Shown here are cross sections of the tubules of newts that have only one set of chromosomes (i.e., they are haploid), or the normal two sets (diploid), or five sets (pentaploid).

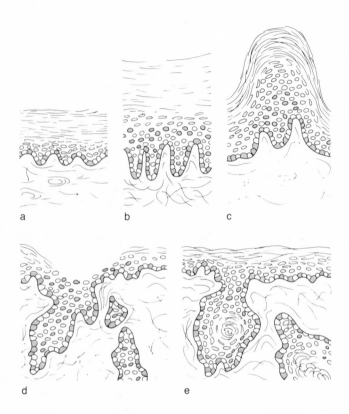

FIGURE 3-6   Varieties of uncontrolled growth of the skin. The pattern of cell multiplication is most easily demonstrated by marking cells with a radioactive precursor of DNA (^{3}H-thymidine); only cells that are about to divide will be marked. In this diagram, such labeled cells are shaded.

(a) *Normal skin.* Cell multiplication is confined to the deepest layer of epithelial cells (the basal cells), which are next to the underlying dermis.

(b) *Psoriasis.* The zone of cell multiplication extends to several layers of cells, so that the rate of production and shedding of cells greatly increases. Here it is as if the primary abnormality lies in the dermis, which seems to be sending out to the overlying epithelium an abnormally strong signal for cell multiplication.

(c) *The common wart.* This is a single family of cells that seem to have slowed down their rate of differentiation, as if they are somewhat freed from the restraints imposed by the dermis.

(d) *Basal-cell carcinoma.* The basal cells have escaped from their normal territorial restraints and are penetrating into the dermis (forming an invasive cancer).

(e) *The squamous-cell carcinoma.* The epithelial cells are invading the dermis but, unlike the basal-cell cancer, they have retained the ability to differentiate into flakes of keratin.

Other minor abnormalities of behavior of melanocytes seem to be unusually common, though this may be simply because the pigment in the melanocyte makes it a very conspicuous cell; for example, we are all familiar with those abnormal families of melanocytes that are called freckles.

These are just some of the disorders of growth shown by epidermis. They demonstrate the most important point that, although there are many ways of releasing cells from whatever forces are normally controlling their multiplication, it is only when cells are freed from the constraints of territoriality that they can form a potentially lethal malignant growth or cancer. Further, as the two common skin cancers show, loss of territoriality can occur in different ways: in each, the exact nature of the defect will determine the exact behavior of the cells, i.e., whether the tumor is benign (noninvasive) or malignant, and whether the cells are likely to spread quickly to distant sites. Therefore it is not sufficient to categorize cancers simply by the organ or type of cell from which they have originated. To be of practical use the classification must be finer, and the way the cancer cells behave should be considered.

A similarly wide range of behavior is shown by the cancers that arise in the sheets of epithelial cells that line the intestine and respiratory tract and form glands such as breast, pancreas, prostate, and so on. These cell types are normally programmed to form systems of cavities and tubes. In the breast, for example, there is strong interaction between adjacent groups of epithelial cells,[21] and between them and the supporting tissue of the breast (equivalent to the dermis and called, as in most organs, the *stroma*). Thus it seems to be the breast stroma that determines to some extent the behavior of the epithelium; for example, the suppression of epithelial growth in the male turns out to be due to the effect of the male hormone, testosterone, upon the stroma rather than directly upon the epithelium itself;[22] similarly, in some species at least, the mammary epithelium will readily turn into apparently normal skin if transplanted onto the surface.[23] At the same time the different lobes of a single mammary gland normally do not invade each other's territory, clearly indicating that different sections of mammary epithelium are sensitive to each other's presence and must therefore be giving forth signals as well as receiving them. The change in behavior of mammary epithelium when it becomes cancerous is shown in Figure 3-7.

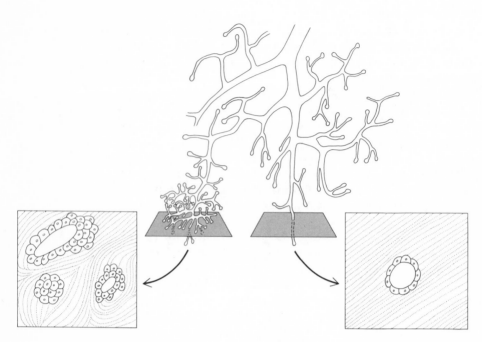

FIGURE 3-7   Early stages in the development of a mammary cancer. The normal mammary epithelium (right) is arranged as an orderly system of branching ducts that tidily fill the available space. The first step in the appearance of a cancer is the formation of a nodule of cells (left) that do not respect the territorial imperatives of adjacent ducts but proliferate uncontrolledly, and invade the surrounding supporting tissues. Sections of the normal and cancerous glands are shown at bottom.

Cancers of glandular epithelia vary in the extent to which they are able to form lobes and ducts. Those that retain this property are called *adenocarcinomas* (literally, "gland" carcinomas) and tend to be rather less malignant than cancers in which the cells show complete loss of order (the so-called *anaplastic,* or undifferentiated carcinomas). It is also possible to classify epithelial cancers according to the response of the accompanying stroma: in some tumors the stromal cells vastly outnumber the epithelial cells, suggesting that one of the qualities of certain cancer cells is the production of much too strong a signal to the neighboring cells. In other tumors there may be little or no stroma.

The variation in behavior of the different cancers that can originate from any single class of cell is reflected not only in differences in the gross and microscopic anatomy of the resulting tumors but also in their response to treatment. Some cancers respond to irradiation, some to hormones, and some to certain cytotoxic drugs. Even though there is no proper explanation for the different behavior and response of different cancers, we can at least deduce from their very variety that each kind of cell can be turned into a cancer cell in several different ways. However, as long as we know so little about the forces normally at work on the healthy cells in a multicellular organism such as man, we may not be able to make much progress in any attempt to categorize the basic defects of the different varieties of cancer cell. Certainly, to date no fundamental theory of carcinogenesis has been proposed that could explain the way different cancers respond to treatment and could be used to develop better drugs. Thus, for the time being, we may do better if we try to determine empirically the causes of each kind of cancer. This brings us to the epidemiology of cancer—the subject of the next chapter.

THE EPIDEMIOLOGY
of CANCER

Judging from the epidemiology of cancer in man, it seems clear that almost all forms of cancer are caused, largely or entirely, by factors in our environment that vary from one place to another and from one generation to the next. Even without knowing what these factors are, we can deduce—in principle at least—that cancer should be a preventable disease.[1]

Historically, the first step in determining the cause of any disease has always been to find out if there is anything, apart from the disease itself, that the sufferers have in common? This was true for the infectious diseases, the various dietary and vitamin deficiencies, the many kinds of "natural" and industrial poisonings, and so on. *A priori*, there is no reason why the same should not be true for the different forms of cancer.

As everyone knows, nearly all forms of cancer are much more common in old people. Before comparing cancer incidence in different geographic and ethnic groups, we have to consider its relation to aging and, in particular, to examine critically the pessimistic idea that most cancer arises from internal causes and therefore cannot be prevented.

Cancer and Aging

It is not generally realized just how steeply cancer incidence rises with age. To take a typical example, the death rate from cancer of the large intestine increases more than one thousand fold between the ages of 30 and 80 (Figure 4-1a); to give an idea of what this means in everyday terms, a factor of one thousand fold is roughly the difference between the chances of ending one's days being struck dead by lightning and of being struck dead by an automobile. Most other forms of cancer show a similar effect of age, and so any ideas we have about the causation of cancer must fit in with the fact that it is predominantly a disease of the old.

Various models have been proposed to account for the way cancer incidence increases with age.[3] They all have in common the concept that a cancer cell arises as the end result of a series of steps that have occurred at some time in the life of the patient. That is the general—intentionally vague—statement. There are many ways of expressing it somewhat more specifically. The simplest—and one that is sufficient for the purposes of this chapter—is to postulate that each cell has several genes that independently restrain it from forming an ever-expanding family of cells, and that a cancer arises when a cell is created in which each of those genes has been inactivated by a separate, independent mutation. Because mutation can occur at any time in the life of a cell or its ancestors, the probability of any particular one of our cells having a mutation in a particular gene will increase in direct

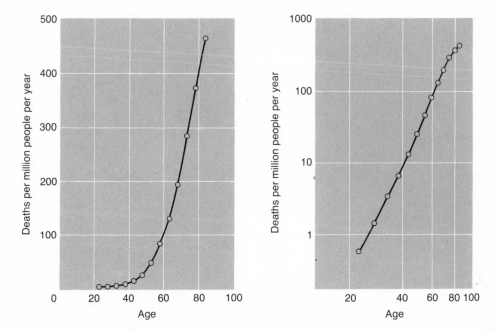

FIGURE 4-1   Annual U.S. death rate from cancer of the large intestine in relation to age, 1968: (a) linear scales; (b) logarithmic scales. [From U.S. Department of Health, Education, and Welfare. *Vital Statistics of the United States*. Volume II. *Mortality*. U.S. Government Printing Office, 1968.]

proportion to our age. So the probability that the cell has mutations in all N of its restraining genes (i.e., has become a cancer) will rise as the Nth power of our age; for example, if the total number, N, of restraining genes were 3, the probability of having cancer would increase as the cube of age. Expressed another way, the logarithm of cancer incidence should be linearly related to the logarithm of our age.* As Figure 4-1b shows, this is indeed approximately correct. Incidentally if such an interpretation were literally true, we could deduce from the slope of the line in the figure that about 6 mutations are needed to produce a cancer of the large intestine.[4]

The mutational model is very attractive because it is the obvious way of describing a change whose salient feature, as we have

---

*To be precise, the risk of having cancer will increase as the Nth power of age and the annual incidence of cancer, being the first derivative, will increase as the $(N-1)$th power of age.

seen, is that it affects all the descendants of a single cell. But it says nothing about the cause of the mutations which, in principle, could be brought on by mutagens in our environment or could occur spontaneously as a result of some inherent imperfection in our cells. Moreover, it is very important to remember that mutational steps are not the only possible basis for such multi-stage models; errors of gene regulation would serve just as well.[5]

Mutation
1. Genetic
2. Epigenetic

Periodically the suggestion is made that the common forms of cancer are just one facet of an overall deliberate program of aging, which has evolved by natural selection and brings some advantage to the species. The argument is as follows: Each species (man included) has evolved to fill efficiently some particular ecological niche. Each niche demands an optimum level of complexity on the part of those who fill it and this complexity determines how much time has to be spent in growing to maturity and therefore how durable the animal must be. Obviously every species must be designed so that the average individual's offspring have sufficient longevity to ensure that several of them can reach sexual maturity and reproduce. But once this level of longevity has been achieved (so the argument goes) it is conceivable that there has been selection, over millions of years, for some aging process that kills off the older animals so that they do not fill up the ecological niche (though one has to admit that there are problematical features to achieving selection for a response which brings absolutely no benefit to the one who is responding). The argument is therefore that man has been designed to die in old age from diseases like cancer and arteriosclerosis and that consequently the causation of these diseases will not have been left to chance factors like environmental carcinogens or oddities of diet, but will prove to depend on intrinsic properties of the cell[6] such as a programmed imprecision in the enzymes that are used for making DNA, RNA, and protein. If this hypothesis were true, obviously we could not hope ever to attain much progress in cancer prevention.

Fortunately the argument is plainly incorrect because it makes the firm prediction that the different groups of people in the world should all have roughly the same overall cancer incidence for any given age and that changes in habits and environment should have little effect on incidence. In fact, as we shall see, these predictions are not fulfilled. Cancer incidence is, to a large extent, determined by environment and so most cancers should, in principle, be preventable.

There is in fact a perfectly good alternative explanation for the changes of aging which does not require that senescence should be actually useful to the species.[7] At any given point in time the most important members of each species are those that have just reached sexual maturity because, of all the animals present, they are the ones with the greatest capacity for increase. So we should expect to find that the animals of each species reach their optimum state at about the time that they become sexually mature; certainly, human resistance to stress is greatest between ages 20 and 30[8] and our annual death rate is at its lowest level at about 15 (Figure 2-1). Now, in certain respects, the price of optimizing the quality of an animal's components for one particular stage in its life is that the quality of these components has to decline from that stage onwards. An example will make this clear. The chief structural protein of our body is collagen.[9] Although it can be made at any time and indeed is the main component of scar tissue, most of our collagen molecules are produced when we are young. They are secreted by cells into the extracellular space and then are slowly cross-linked to produce the tough strong fibers that give our tissues and organs their shape and physical strength. The process of cross-linking is accomplished by extracellular enzymes and continues throughout our whole life in such a steady, regular manner that it is possible to determine people's age to within about five years simply by testing a sample of their collagen.[10] Because cross-linking never stops, our collagen goes through a period of maximum strength and then becomes increasingly brittle as we get older. Similar changes occur in other components. One most easily visible to the naked eye is the decline in elasticity and thickness (cellularity) of our skin, but it is plain that other, microscopic changes are also occurring throughout all the cells of the body; and it is easy to imagine that even such a complex process as the development of our nervous system is timed to culminate at just about the same stage as our collagen.

These alterations are essentially uniform; pinch into a fold any part of an old person's skin and you will see that the loss of elasticity does not vary from one area to another. It is not therefore a rare random process like mutation, but a regular program. Furthermore, this program could have arisen without there ever having been positive selection for any decline in durability with age, but simply as a consequence of the need to produce an optimum product.

At the same time as we undergo this kind of uniform aging, we also acquire scattered patchy abnormalities that, because they seem to represent individual families of cells, are probably due to chance random mutations. For example, the commonest cause of death in the United States is atheroma of the arteries. This is the condition in which thickened patches (atheromatous plaques) develop in the walls of the arteries, and death occurs when there is obstruction of one of the few small arteries in the body that are essential for life, namely the arteries supplying the heart and brain. Recent studies of X-chromosome mosaics have shown that each atheromatous plaque is apparently a single family of abnormal cells,[11] i.e., that we are dealing here, as in the case of cancer, with a disease that originates in single cells, perhaps as the result of mutation.[12]

Even though atheroma and cancer make up such a large proportion of the deaths in old age, and now amount to two-thirds of all deaths in the United States (see Table 2-1), it does not follow automatically that these diseases should be classed as yet another manifestation of the uniform, inexorable processes of senescence. If they are caused by random mutations, these mutations could be due to some programmed imprecision in the way cells handle their genetic material, like the imprecision in handling collagen; but they could just as easily be due to external factors. In order to determine the cause of diseases like atheroma and cancer, we must resort to epidemiology.

The Epidemiology of Cancer

It is about 170 years since the first plan was proposed for determining the causes of cancer by studying its incidence in relation to such factors as occupation, sex, marital status, and so on.[13] But the appropriate statistical methods were not developed until the middle of the 19th century, and it was not until after World War I that cancer registries were set up in various Western countries. Only in the last 25 years has there been a concerted effort to collect statistics for many different regions of the world, and for a set of populations selected to represent as wide a range of environments and life styles as possible. From all this work a rough idea has emerged of how the incidence of cancer (and the resulting death rate) varies in different countries and social groups and how it changes as people alter their habits or move from one country to another.

Worldwide Variation in the Incidence of Cancer

The industrial nations now routinely collect statistics for the various forms of mortality including that due to cancer. In addition about 100 special cancer registries, scattered throughout the world, continually record the incidence of cancer for particular limited populations (i.e., the number of new cases arising each year).[14] Even a cursory glance at this huge compilation of data reveals that cancer incidence (and mortality) varies greatly from one country to another. Cancer of the liver is the commonest cancer among men in Mozambique but is rare in Europe and the United States, whereas the opposite is true for cancer of the lung; cancer of the bladder is common in Egypt, and cancer of the stomach is especially common in Japan; skin cancer is common in sunny areas. (It is worth mentioning that people have looked for some form of cancer that has a constant incidence in all populations and so can be used as a standard for checking the reliability of the different cancer registries; although there is a rare form of cancer of the kidney in childhood that is in this category,[15] the significant fact is that this standard has been hard to find.)

Table 4-1 shows how greatly the incidence of the common cancers varies from one country to another. It has been calculated that an imaginary population, which had the lowest recorded rate for each kind of cancer, would enjoy a cancer incidence about one-tenth of that in most Western countries;[16] for that imaginary population, cancer would not be a major cause of death. There is, however, an unavoidable ambiguity in this kind of information, because it does not distinguish between the effects of environment and those of genetic constitution. It is crucial therefore to find out whether the differences in cancer incidence, from one population to another, are due to potentially alterable environmental factors, or to unalterable genetic variation.

If the subject of study were an experimental animal, the next step in the analysis would be to carry out either a breeding experiment or a study of the effects of altering the environment. However, thanks to the speed of change in the modern industrial state and the mass migrations that reflect the changing fortunes of

TABLE 4-1   Variation in incidence of the common cancers

Type of cancer	Region of highest incidence	Risk up to age 75 (%)	Range of variation*	Region of lowest incidence
Men				
Skin	Queensland	Over 20	Over 200	Bombay
Esophagus	Northeast Iran	20	300	Nigeria
Lung	Great Britain	11	35	Nigeria
Stomach	Japan	11	25	Uganda
Liver	Mozambique	8	70	Norway
Prostate	U.S. (Blacks)	7	30	Japan
Colon	Connecticut	3	10	Nigeria
Mouth	India	Over 2	Over 25	Denmark
Rectum	Denmark	2	20	Nigeria
Bladder	Connecticut	2	4	Japan
Women				
Cervix	Colombia	10	15	Israel (Jews)
Breast	Connecticut	7	15	Uganda

SOURCE R. Doll. "Strategy for detection of cancer hazards to man." *Nature* **265,** 589–596 (1977).

*The highest incidence observed in any country divided by the lowest observed incidence.

nations and the propensity of man to persecute minorities, many inadvertent experiments have been carried out.

Change in Incidence with Time

If we were living in the Middle Ages or earlier, when human customs did not alter much from one century to the next, we could not hope to observe any effects of environment on cancer incidence simply by looking for fluctuations in incidence with time. As it is, we live in a world devoted to innovation and change and one of the consequences is a changing pattern of cancer incidence. This class of information is very important because each large group of people can be considered to have a constant genetic constitution from one generation to the next. Any significant trend in the incidence of some cancer must therefore represent the effect of some change in environment—an effect over which we can in principle exercise control. Two examples stand out (Figure 4-2).

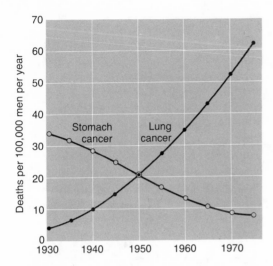

FIGURE 4-2   The death rate from stomach cancer and lung cancer in U.S. males since 1930. The values shown in this figure have been standardized for a population with an unchanging age distribution and have been brought up to date by the inclusion of estimated death rates that were published by the American Cancer Society. [Data after T. Gordon, M. Crittenden, and W. Haenszel. *Cancer Mortality Trends in the United States, 1930–1955.* Natn. Cancer Inst. Monograph 6, 131–350, 1961; F. Burbank. *Patterns in cancer mortality in the United States; 1950–1967.* Natn. Cancer Inst. Monograph *33,* 1971.]

Throughout this century the incidence of cancer of the lung has steadily increased, so that by now in many Western countries it is the commonest of all cancers. Yet in the 19th century it was a rare diagnosis. From the very beginning of the increase, some people thought it was probably due to tobacco; but others considered it to be not an actual increase but merely a reflection of changing fashions of diagnosis. What confused people at first was the conspicuous lack of correlation between a nation's cigarette consumption (a readily accessible statistic) and its lung cancer rate. The discrepancy was resolved once it was realized that there is roughly a 20-year interval between the time at which a group of people start to smoke and the time that they show a measurable increase in lung cancer (but see later chapters for a more detailed discussion of the time course of carcinogenesis); when corrected for this effect, the correlation becomes very good (Figure 4-3). A separate, but equally persuasive argument for the role of cigarettes is the way in which both cigarette smoking and lung cancer

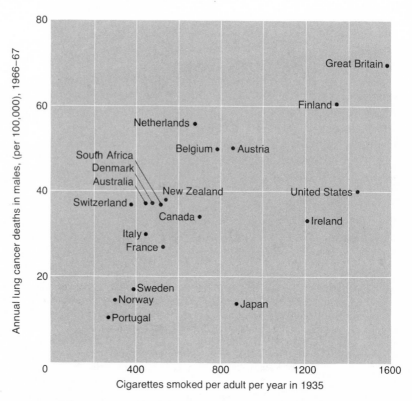

FIGURE 4-3   Relation between cigarette consumption and each nation's
annual deaths from lung cancer 30 years later. [Data after N. Wald, personal
communication. This figure is also reproduced in E. L. Wynder and S. Hecht,
Eds., *UICC Technical Report Series* **25**, 1976.]

increased for men long before they increased for women (Figure
4-4); it could have been argued that the rise in lung cancer was
due to changing accuracy or fashions in diagnosis, but it is hardly
possible to believe in a diagnostic bias that for a period of 50
years applied only to male patients. Cancer of the lung is the most
spectacular example in which the cause of a cancer has been
determined by studying the way incidence changes with time
(i.e., within groups which effectively have an unchanging genetic
make-up). Indeed, in retrospect, it is almost as if Western societies
had set out to conduct a vast and fairly well controlled experiment in carcinogenesis bringing about several million deaths and
using their own people as the experimental animals.

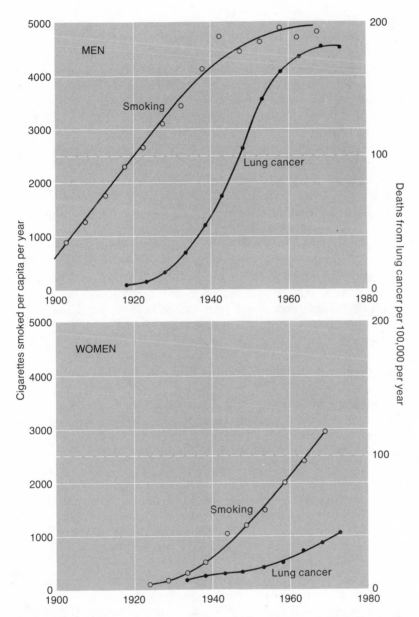

FIGURE 4-4   Relation between smoking and the subsequent rise in the death rate from lung cancer, for men and women in England. [After Royal College of Physicians, *Smoking and Health Now,* Pitman Medical and Scientific Publishing Company, 1971.]

The other example, cancer of the stomach, is interesting because its incidence has changed almost as markedly as that of cancer of the lung but in the opposite direction; since 1930, the annual death rate in the United States has dropped about fivefold. The change cannot be attributed to improved treatment, because the five-year survival rate for this cancer is still only about 10%. The cause of the change is completely unknown. It is perhaps typical of the way mankind organizes its affairs that we have inadvertently progressed a long way towards preventing one major form of cancer, whereas we seem quite incapable of steeling ourselves to abolish another when we have discovered its cause.

Many other common forms of cancer have, in the course of time, shown a significant but smaller shift in frequency.[17] For example, in the United States the death rates from cancer of the pancreas and the nervous sytem have risen four- to fivefold in the past 40 years; the leukemias increased about threefold between 1930 and 1950 but have stayed fairly constant since then; and the death rate from cancer of the cervix has been falling since 1950. The cause of these changes is not known.

Variation in Incidence among Different Social Groups

Within the United States the total death rate from all forms of cancer varies significantly from state to state.[18] The highest rates tend to be in states in the northeast (New York, Connecticut, Massachusetts, and Rhode Island) which are all about 10% above the national average; the lowest are in the mountain states of Utah, Wyoming, and Idaho, where the overall rate is about 25% below average. The rates for the individual cancers often vary more than this, the extremes covering a twofold range for certain cancers. The implication is that about a third of the cancer deaths in the high-risk states would not have occurred if the victims had lived in the West.

The effect of other environmental factors is seen if we divide the population of the United States according to degree of affluence (using their level of education as a convenient estimator of socioeconomic level). Of the principal varieties of cancer, only cancer of the breast and prostate are commoner among the rich; the others tend to be commoner among the poor, who therefore have a somewhat higher overall death rate from cancer than the rich (Table 4-2). These statistics prompt the obvious thought that

TABLE 4-2   Age-adjusted* death rates from certain types of cancer for people in the U.S. over the age of 25, according to level of education

Cancer Site	Death rate (ratio to death rates among college graduates)		
	Persons with less than 8 years of school	Persons with 8 years of school	High school graduates
Males			
Stomach	2.0	1.9	1.8
Lung	1.6	1.4	1.4
Prostate	0.5	0.5	0.5
All sites	1.1	1.1	1.0
Females			
Stomach	2.7	2.3	2.1
Large intestine	1.3	1.5	1.4
Uterus and ovary	1.5	1.3	1.3
Breast	0.7	0.9	0.9
All sites	1.1	1.1	1.1

SOURCE   A. M. Lilienfeld, M. L. Levin and I. I. Kessler. Cancer in the United States. Harvard University Press, Cambridge, Mass (1972)

*Note on age-adjusted death rates. When two countries are to be compared that have populations with different age distributions, the death rates are measured in each 5 year age-group in each population. From these rates it is then possible to calculate what would have been the overall death rate in each country if its population had shown the same age distribution as, for example, the United States as a whole. This correction is essential for any disease like cancer, that has an incidence which is closely related to age.

most forms of cancer seem to be brought on by factors which are concentrated in industrialized urban areas and to which the poor are more exposed than the rich—such as air pollution, peculiarities of diet, or even that shadowy specter called stress.

For most cancers, it should be possible to get some idea about the factor or factors responsible by conducting a detailed survey of all the easily measured variables in the lives of the populations of a few appropriate regions. Two examples will demonstrate the kind of result that can be obtained. Within a single nation like the United States cancer of the large intestine is somewhat commoner among the poor, but a comparison of different nations reveals that this cancer is plainly commoner in the wealthier countries. In seeking the cause, it has seemed natural to examine diet just as it seemed reasonable, when investigating lung cancer, to look for an inhaled carcinogen. A detailed analysis of the habits of many nations suggests that the most likely cause is a high level of meat in the diet, in particular beef, or a low intake of cereals (Figure 4-5). One proposal is that various carcinogens are created within the large intestine by bacterial decomposition of certain bile sterols and that these are present in greater quantities and

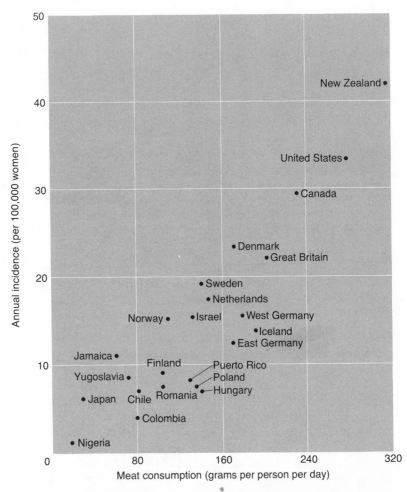

FIGURE 4-5   The age-adjusted incidence of cancer of the colon in the women of different nations, in relation to average meat consumption. [After B. Armstrong and R. Doll. *Int. J. Cancer* 15, 617–631 (1975).]

remain there for a longer time if the diet contains a lot of meat and little roughage.[19]

Other factors apart from diet and effects of industrialization distinguish one social group from another. For example, the incidence of breast cancer varies greatly among different nations and different social groups within a single nation. As we might guess, one of the decisive factors is related to reproductive history: namely, it turns out the sooner a woman has her first child, the less likely is she in later life to develop breast cancer (Figure 4-6). The explanation may lie in the rather peculiar behavior of breast epithelium in relation to pregnancy,[20] but whatever the reason we see that the incidence of breast cancer is being decisively influenced by what might loosely be called our life style.

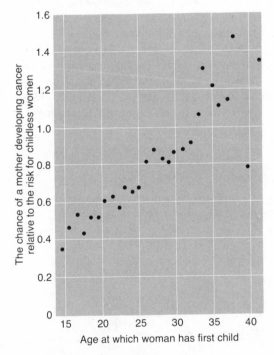

FIGURE 4-6   The chance that a woman develops breast cancer at some time in her life is lowest for those women who bore their first child when they were very young. This chance increases steadily the longer the first child bearing is postponed. [After B. MacMahon, P. Cole, and J. Brown. *J. Natn. Cancer Inst.* **50,** 21–42 (1973).]

Studies on Migrants

The case for believing that habits, diet, and environment are decisive would be greatly strengthened if we could deliberately manipulate people's lives. Short-term controlled experiments have been carried out on the effects of diet on heart disease, in which the subjects have been the inmates of a pair of mental homes, for example. But there would be strong ethical (and practical) barriers to exposing people deliberately and for a long period to any factor thought to cause cancer. Fortunately, people do the experiments themselves. Groups migrate from one country to another, or adopt new habits through the exigencies of war or the demands of religion. By studying them we can compare to some extent the contributions of genetic and nongenetic factors, and even get some idea of the time course of human carcinogenesis.

For example, in Japan cancer of the stomach is much more common than it is in the United States, but cancers of the large intestine, breast, and prostate are less common. When the Japanese emigrate to the United States, these differences decline within a generation or two (Table 4-3). Because the immigrants and their children tend to marry within the group, the change in incidence must be caused by the changed environment rather than by genetic factors;[21] (the argument requires the reasonable

TABLE 4-3   Age-adjusted death rates for various cancers observed among male Japanese in Japan, male Japanese immigrants to California, and these immigrants' sons born in California. The results are expressed as the ratio of the number of deaths that occurred, divided by the number that would have been expected in a similar group of Californian Caucasians.

Cancer site	Death rates (ratio to death rates in California whites)		
	Japanese in Japan	Japanese immigrants to California	Sons of Japanese immigrants
Stomach	6.5	4.6	3.0
Liver	3.7	2.1	2.2
Colon	0.2	0.8	0.9
Prostate	0.1	0.5	1.0

SOURCE   P. Buell and J. E. Dunn. Cancer mortality among Japanese Issei and Nisei of California. *Cancer* 18, 656–664 (1965).

assumption that the Japanese who migrate are typical of the population as a whole, and are not a particular subgroup with a genetic constitution that prompts them to migrate to a country where the inhabitants have a cancer incidence like their own). The data in the table show that the incidence of the various cancers takes rather more than one generation to reach levels typical of the United States; we may therefore conclude that some of the causative agents must be factors such as diet, that tend to persist as part of the cultural heritage, rather than others such as air pollution, which tend to be the same for everyone.

Similarly, the Jews who migrated to Israel from Europe or the United States exhibit a cancer incidence that is typical for their country of origin, but their children born in Israel have a much lower incidence of almost all kinds of cancer and in this respect have become more like the indigenous Jewish and Arab populations and the Jewish migrants from Asia and Africa (Table 4-4). Although to some extent these migrants, like the Japanese migrants to California, will have persisted with the habits and customs of their countries of origin, many of them migrated as children and will presumably have adopted the local habits. If that is correct, we are forced to conclude that human carcinogenesis is commonly a very long and gradual process: the child in central Europe is exposed to the European carcinogen in youth, migrates to Israel and, many years later, develops the resultant cancer. This is a most important conclusion and will be discussed further in Chapter 9.

TABLE 4-4 The overall age-adjusted incidence rate for all forms of cancer, among the four main groups in Israel in 1961–1965, compared to the rate in the U.S.

Group	Population	Annual Incidence per 100,000	
		Males	Females
Non-Jews (mostly Arabs)	140,000	179	93
Jews born in Israel	425,000	193	195
Jews born in Africa or elsewhere in Asia	291,000	208	167
Jews born in the U.S. or Europe	352,000	294	313
General U.S. population		300–400	300–400

SOURCE   R. Doll, C. Muir and J. Waterhouse. Cancer incidence in five continents. UICC. Springer-Verlag, Berlin. (1970)

Genetic Factors

On general principles we should expect to find that our susceptibility to cancer, like our other qualities, is influenced to some
extent by our genetic constitution. Certainly, it has been possible
by selective breeding to develop many lines of mice that have a
very high incidence of various forms of cancer.[22] There are various
reasons for studying the genetics of cancer. One is that we would
like to know if we can identify those families with an abnormally
high risk of developing cancer, because we could then advise
them on what habits or occupations to avoid that increase the
risk of getting the kind of cancer to which they have an inherited
susceptibility, and we could also check them regularly in the hope
of achieving earlier treatment.

Given the very strong influence of habits and environment
upon the incidence of each kind of cancer, it is to be expected that
the members of any one family will inevitably tend to be more
like each other in their cancer experience than they are like the
population at large. For example, at first sight it may seem surprising that not only do the sisters of women with cancer of the
cervix have a raised incidence of the same cancer, but their
fathers turn out to have a significantly increased incidence of
cancer of the esophagus;[23] however, the reason is simply that both
kinds of cancer are commonest among one particular sector of the
populace, namely the poor.

Nevertheless, it is possible to detect a genuine familial tendency for some of the major varieties of cancer. For example,
cancer of the breast is about three times commoner in both paternal and maternal female relatives of breast cancer patients
than in the general population or in the relatives of patients with
other forms of cancer.[24] Similarly, cancer of the stomach and large
intestine are somewhat commoner in the relatives of patients.
There is, however, no evidence that many families have a
heightened susceptibility to all forms of cancer in general.[25] Each
of the major cancers behaves almost as an independent entity;
with few exceptions, people who have been successfully treated
for one cancer are then neither more nor less likely in subsequent
years to come down with a second, different variety.[26]

In principle, the best way of measuring the contribution of genetic constitution is by determining the extent to which identical
(*monozygotic*) twins are more like each other than are nonidentical (*dizygotic*) twins. Unfortunately it is not easy to assemble

large numbers of suitable twins: cancer is a disease of old age, twins have a higher infant mortality than single births, and it is not often that both twins survive to an age where they are at all likely to have cancer. However several such surveys have been carried out. The general conclusion is that identical twins are not much more alike in the cancers they suffer than are nonidentical twins.[27] Therefore in man the contribution of genetics seems to be rather slight for the common forms of cancer, at least when compared to the contribution of envirionment.

So far we have been thinking about inherited characteristics that raise susceptibility. One trait that decreases susceptibility is pigmentation. Cancer of the skin is much less common in people who are dark complexioned, presumably because they are better protected against ultraviolet light.[28] A rather similar effect has been proposed for one of the enzymes that act on certain carcinogens (see p. 99); it has been suggested that those people who have inherited the trait for synthesizing only a small quantity of the enzyme arylhydrocarbon hydroxylase are much less susceptible to the carcinogenic effect of cigarettes and have a lower lung cancer rate than might be expected from their smoking habits,[29] (although other nongenetic factors also influence the level of this enzyme).[30]

There is another, academic reason for being interested in the genetics of cancer. Several rare inherited diseases of man are associated with certain unusual cancers, and these give us a hint about the steps that can contribute to the formation of a cancer.[31] For example, one rare disease called xeroderma pigmentosum causes the patient's skin to be exceptionally sensitive to sunlight and the skin usually develops multiple cancers as a result; the basic defect, which is inherited as a simple Mendelian recessive (see p. 80), turns out to be in the enzymes that repair DNA damaged by ultraviolet light (see p. 85), and so this finding supports the idea that cancer can result from mutation. These rare inherited cancers reveal more about the underlying mechanisms of carcinogenesis than they do about the causes of the common cancers.

The Epidemiology of Certain Rare Occupational Cancers

Any discussion of the epidemiology of cancer would be incomplete without some mention of the special cancers associated with various industries. Even collectively, the occupational cancers are not large in number, but they demonstrate how it is often possible to guess the cause of a cancer even when there are few cases to go on, and they also provide some of the few successful contributions of cancer research to preventive medicine.

The most famous example, cancer of the scrotum in chimney sweeps, was described 200 years ago, and this report (along with the slightly earlier one on cancer of the nose in snuff-takers) was the first positive identification of the cause of any cancer. The account is unusually vivid.

> The fate of these people seems singularly hard; in their early infancy, they are most frequently treated with great brutality, and almost starved with cold and hunger; they are thrust up narrow, and sometimes hot chimneys, where they are bruised, burned, and almost suffocated; and when they get to puberty, become peculiarly liable to a most noisome, painful, and fatal disease. Of this last circumstance there is not the least doubt, though perhaps it may not have been sufficiently attended to, to make it generally known.[32]

The link could be made because the cancer was common in sweeps and virtually unknown in the rest of the population (until the 1850s, when mineral oils began to replace animal oils for lubricating machines, probably the only potent chemical carcinogen for skin that people came into contact with was soot from chimneys).

Following that classic example, the list of unusual cancers with readily identifiable causes has steadily risen. Some are due to outlandish habits (chewing tobacco, smoking cigars with the burning end held inside one's mouth, keeping warm by holding a burning brazier against one's stomach, and so on), and some are due to particular occupational hazards.

The development of the chemistry of coal-tar derivatives from about 1850 onwards and the discovery of the synthetic dyes triggered the sudden birth of new industries in which workers were exposed to large quantities of compounds that in time proved to be extremely carcinogenic. For example, the compound 2-naphthylamine can be the starting material for the synthesis of many dyes, and its large-scale production began in Germany in about 1890. The first crop of bladder cancers associated with its use was reported five years later, but a protracted argument then ensued about the causal connection because cancer of the bladder is not uncommon in the population at large, and so in several countries it was not for another 50 years that large-scale produc-

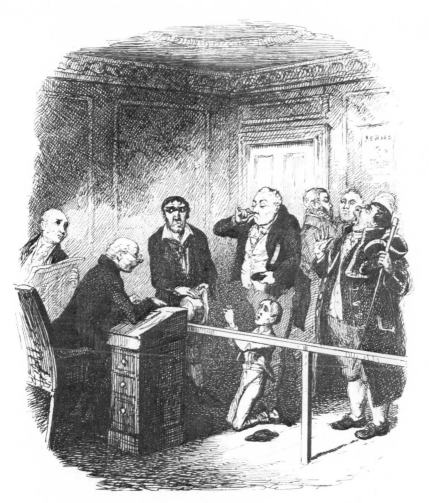

FIGURE 4-7   Oliver escapes being bound apprentice to the sweep. [From Charles Dickens, *The Adventures of Oliver Twist*, Chapman and Hall, 1874.]

tion was brought to a halt.[33] Although the total number of deaths from bladder cancer caused by 2-naphthylamine in the whole world, in the course of a period of 50 years, is probably lower than the number of deaths from lung cancer in the United States each week, it is a very instructive example. Thus the cancer usually appears after an interval of many years, but because it can eventually affect almost all the workers who were heavily exposed (Figure 4-8), there is no indication that any people are genetically

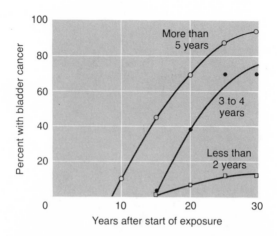

FIGURE 4-8   The time of appearance of bladder cancer in a group of 78 men exposed to 2-naphthylamine. The men are divided into three groups, according to total duration of their exposure. [After M.H.C. Williams, "Occupational tumors of the bladder in cancer." In R. W. Raven, ed., *Cancer*, Vol. III. Butterworth (1958).]

insusceptible; even so, in one sense 2-naphthylamine is just barely a carcinogen in man, because the bladder seems to be the only tissue that is susceptible and, but for this one organ's susceptibility, we could presumably handle large quantities with impunity. We see here two of the characteristic features of the carcinogenic process—the lengthy interval between initial stimulus and final response, and the apparent difficulty in predicting what the actual response to any carcinogen is going to be. Both these features will be discussed further in later chapters.

Certain occupational cancers demonstrate another important feature of carcinogenesis, namely that the production of a cancer may depend not on any single agent but on the interaction of separate factors. For example, asbestos dust is very irritating to the lung and causes the chronic disabling disease called asbestosis; it can also cause lung cancer. However, further analysis has revealed that these cancers arise almost exclusively in people exposed to asbestos dust who also smoke.[34] As we shall see in Chapter 7, several procedures are carcinogenic in experimental animals only if preceded by treatment with another agent.

Because of these few spectacular examples of occupational cancers, it has recently become fashionable to blame industry for all the other forms of cancer. And as each new report comes out that yet another chemical product has been shown to be carcinogenic and should therefore be removed from the market, more and more people probably become more and more convinced that science lies at the root of all our troubles. In fact, with the exception of lung cancer, all the common cancers have been common since the 19th century. For example, in the United States there has been little change in the incidence and death rate from cancer as a whole in the last 30 years during which time the annual production of pesticides, synthetic rubber, and plastics has risen more than 100-fold (Figure 4-9). Thus, although some of these chemicals may cause cancer in the future, it does not seem that industry can be made the scapegoat for the cancers that are common at the moment.

The Clustering of Cancer Cases

For a variety of reasons, there has been great pressure to investigate the possible role of viruses in human cancer, and this has led to the search for evidence that cancer can be spread by contact and will be found often to occur in clusters of cases. One incentive is that the conquest of infectious diseases lies within existing technology, whereas the prevention or specific treatment of the kinds of aberration of growth control shown by most cancers takes us into unknown territory. In addition, the mechanism of viral carcinogenesis is something that can be investigated by the existing procedures of molecular biology which were developed for studying bacterial cells and their viruses, whereas the mechanisms of chemical carcinogenesis are thought, rightly or wrongly, to be less accessible. For these reasons, viral carcinogenesis has probably received somewhat more attention than it deserves.

Several forms of cancer in animals are due to infective agents. To give just a few examples, the cause of leukemia in cats, or at least one of the factors contributing to the disease, is infection by a virus (see p. 111).[35] There are two very unusual infective cancers of dogs, one due to a parasitic worm that causes a sarcoma of the esophagus,[36] and the other apparently due to a most extraordinary cancer cell that has acquired the ability to spread among dogs as a venereal disease.[37] Flocks of chickens can suffer outbreaks of a leukemia-like disease that is due to a virus, and they may be protected from it by vaccination.[38] And various inbred strains of mice exhibit a high incidence of leukemia or mammary cancer, caused in part by the presence of a virus.

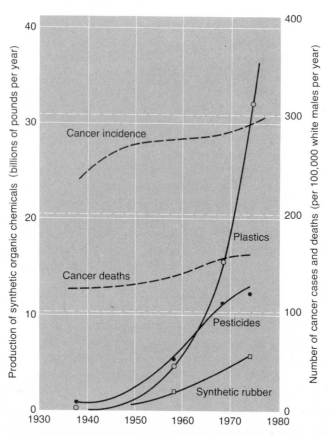

FIGURE 4-9   The production of plastics, pesticides and synthetic rubber have risen precipitously in the United States since World War II. In contrast, the age-adjusted incidence of cancer and resulting death rates have not changed greatly; the slow increase for white males, shown here, is due largely to the increase in lung cancer in smokers. [After R. H. Harris, T. Page, and N. A. Reiches, "Carcinogenic hazards of organic chemicals in drinking water." In H. H. Hiatt, J. D. Watson, and J. A. Winsten, *Origins of Human Cancer*, pp. 309–330, Cold Spring Harbor Laboratory (1977).]

The epidemiological evidence for spread of cancer from one human being to another (so-called "horizontal" transmission, as opposed to the "vertical" transmission of viruses that can occur from parent to child) is rather scant. The obstacle to obtaining more conclusive information is that any infective agent which causes cancer will probably have an incubation period of several years and, what is worse, will probably spread indirectly by way of intermediaries who act as carriers but do not themselves suffer the disease; certainly this seems to be true for feline leukemia, which is one of the two or three clear examples of a horizontally transmitted cancer in animals.

One human cancer for which there is some evidence of horizontal transmission is cancer of the cervix. This cancer is virtually unknown in nuns and is most common in women who have had several sexual partners.[39] Also its incidence is higher in the wives of previously married men if a former wife had cancer of the cervix.[40] There is evidence therefore that it is a venereally transmitted disease, perhaps due to infection by one of the herpesviruses.[41]

There have been numerous reports that certain cancers, in particular leukemia and Hodgkin's disease (a complex cancer affecting several classes of cell present in lymph glands), can occur in clusters of individuals who are interrelated, not by occupation or habits, but by a history of social contact, either directly or through an intermediary. One of the most famous examples was that of an apparent outbreak of Hodgkin's disease in Albany, New York, spread over more than 10 years among a group of schoolchildren and their friends and relatives.[42] This conclusion, however, has been hotly debated.[43] It is extremely difficult to be sure that any such cluster of cases has not occurred as a result of chance alone, especially since fortuitous clusters, like freak hands at bridge, attract attention whereas a normal incidence of cases does not. Furthermore, even if we could be sure that one particular township had a significant excess of cases (i.e., more than would be expected to occur by chance alone in any one of the hundreds of townships in the United States), we would still have to establish that the cases were genuinely related to each other by direct or indirect contact; after all, any two people in the same town will, if they come from the same socioeconomic group, probably have some friend in common.*

---

*An interesting exercise in statistical reasoning comes in here. Imagine that you are an onlooker at a bridge game and notice that on a couple of occasions one of the players has all four aces. You suspect that he is cheating and decide to keep a tally of his hands. You may well do him an injustice, however, if you include in your final reckoning the two hands that made you single him out for attention; they are the stimulus for your hypothesis that he cheats, but the "experiment" to test your hypothesis must not include them. Similarly, the one or two cases of a rare disease that make a doctor wonder if his community is the center of an outbreak must be excluded from the statistical analysis of the incidence of the disease within the community.

If it is difficult to establish that a fairly rare condition like Hodgkin's disease can spread horizontally, the corollary is also true: we could easily be failing to notice spread even if it were occurring. This is especially likely for diseases in which the incubation period after infection is long and variable. Recently certain virus diseases have been demonstrated for which the incubation period is a sizeable fraction of the host's lifespan [44] Most of them have been observed when they have suddenly spread among isolated groups of susceptible animals, such as flocks of sheep or primitive tribes. Obviously a slow epidemic spreading through a typically mobile Western society would be much harder to detect.

One cancer in which clustering has been demonstrated is a condition affecting the lymph glands in the head and neck, called

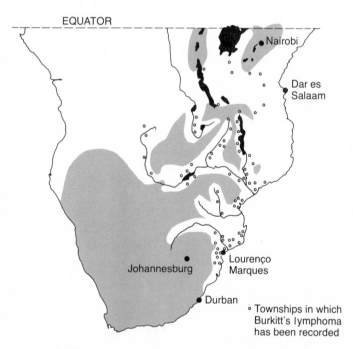

FIGURE 4-10   The distribution of Burkitt's lymphoma. This rare cancer, which afflicts children in Africa, does not occur in regions where the temperature regularly drops below 64°F (gray areas). This suggests that it is transmitted by mosquitoes. The most likely agent is chronic malaria, perhaps in some association with EB virus which, in Africa, is almost invariably present in children from an early age. [After D. Burkitt, Cancer **16**, 379–386 (1962).]

Burkitt's lymphoma. It is a rare disease of children in Africa and occurs even less frequently elsewhere. Like some of the leukemias, it is associated with one particular chromosomal rearrangement[45] which, in Africa, seems to be caused by some complex interaction between chronic malaria and a viral infection.[46] As might be expected, it has attracted a lot of attention as part of the general campaign to establish viruses as significant causes of cancer, although recent evidence suggests that its immediate, precipitating cause is malaria rather than a virus.[47]

Summary

We have seen in this chapter how epidemiology gives us some idea about the causes of human cancer. One or two agents have been positively identified (such as tobacco products and certain industrial chemicals), but for most of the common cancers the analysis is still far from complete. Nevertheless it seems likely that as the epidemiology of cancer eventually becomes understood in much greater detail we will be able to identify the main carcinogenic factors in our lives.

An alternative view is that the factors causing most cancers will be found to be either indecipherable or so closely tied to our chosen lifestyle that the prevention of cancer by removing them is absolutely out of the question. If this turns out to be correct, we will have to approach the cancer problem in some other way, and that is really what the rest of this book is about.

THE EARLY HISTORY
of CANCER RESEARCH

Biology and cancer research have developed together. Invariably, at each stage, the characteristics of the cancer cell have been ascribed to some defect in whatever branch of biology happens at the time to be fashionable and exciting; today it is molecular genetics. Even if the various advances in biology have not thus far provided the key to understanding cancer, they have at least provided an explanation for some of the puzzling phenomena discovered by people doing cancer research.

Cancer is not uncommon in domesticated animals. In the 19th century many attempts were made to transplant pieces of cancerous tissue from one animal to another.[1] Most of the experiments failed because, as we now know, the cells of each animal carry special proteins on their surface that distinguish them from any other animal's cells. This is why, for example, a piece of our skin, if grafted on to someone else, will evoke an immune response and be rejected. These surface components of cells, which are called histocompatibility antigens, are found in all higher animals and effectively prevent the casual accidental spread of cells from one animal to another (though it is not at all clear that this is why they are present). Fortunately, there are a few exceptions to the embargo on transplantation. Our histocompatibility antigens are inherited from our parents, and so grafts will "take" perfectly between identical twins or between the members of any intensely inbred population. Also, graft rejection is most powerful for skin and much less effective for internal organs, so that it is necessary to produce only a slight depression of the immune system in order to make a patient capable of tolerating a kidney transplant. Fortunately, our red blood cells use a much cruder system to identify themselves and so it is easy to find matching cells for blood transfusion. However, none of this was known in the 19th century, and the earliest experiments met with failure.

One of the first successes, in the 1870s, was with a canine sarcoma that proved to be readily transplantable.[2] This was probably the very peculiar sarcoma of dogs mentioned earlier, which is due to a cell that has lost or somehow masked its histocompatibility antigens and is, to this day, spreading among dogs as a venereal disease. But there were also occasional reports of the transplantation of tumors in rats.

In many of the tumors that proved to be transplantable the active component being transferred was not the actual cells but a virus, so that here too no histocompatibility barrier existed. For instance, in the 1890s the common human wart—the kind that children often have on their hands and knees—was shown to be transplantable, and in 1907 the active principle was demonstrated in cell-free extracts. Shortly afterwards the same was found to be true for a leukemia and a sarcoma of chickens. In the case of the chicken sarcoma it now seems likely that, as a result of the repeated attempts to transfer the tumor from one chicken to another across the histocompatibility barrier, the "information" needed to make cells cancerous was transferred to a virus that happened to be present in the chickens; this interesting idea will be discussed in a later chapter (p. 118). For other tumors, the selection pressure caused the cancer cells to lose most of their histocompatibility antigens.

Like the transplantation of spontaneous tumors, the experimental production of cancers in animals proved to be unexpectedly difficult. The first industrial cancers observed in man were the skin cancers caused by prolonged exposure to soot, tar, and various mineral oils, and so it was natural for people to try to produce the same kinds of tumors in animals. Unfortunately they made two mistakes. They did not realize that cancer would arise only after prolonged exposure to tar, and they tended to stop their experiments too soon; second, they elected to do their experiments on dogs and rats—both unlucky choices since neither species is nearly as susceptible as man to this kind of carcinogenesis, perhaps simply because their skin is much thicker. So it was not until 1915 that the first cancer was induced experimentally, by applying tar repeatedly to the ears of rabbits over a period of many months.[3] The long time required for carcinogenesis seems to be central to the problem of cancer, and the subject will come up repeatedly throughout the rest of the book.

After that work, other ways of producing cancer in animals were discovered. Also at about the same time, various highly inbred lines of mice became available that had been selected for a particularly high (or low) spontaneous incidence of leukemia or mammary cancer.[4] So the mouse acquired the invidious status of being the most convenient animal for experimental cancer research. One common procedure is illustrated in Figure 5-1.

From the very outset, the obvious interpretation of carcinogenesis was that it represented an irreversible change in the inherited characteristics of a cell (i.e., what we would now call the *mutation of genes*, though the word *gene* was not invented until well into the 20th century).[5] Indeed, the foundations of the science of genetics were being laid down at the same time as much of this work was being done, and so it was natural to link the two subjects together. There was, however, a disappointing lack of coherence in the whole field of cancer research, and no underlying rules governing the response to carcinogens seemed to exist. One species would be sensitive to one carcinogen but not another, and a given carcinogen such as 2-naphthylamine would single out one

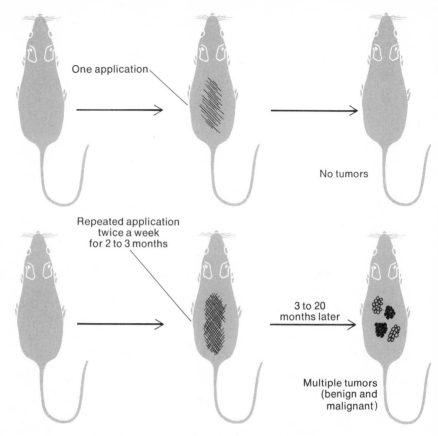

FIGURE 5-1   The appearance of skin tumors in mice after repeated local application of a carcinogen such as coal tar or cigarette smoke condensate.

particular tissue such as the bladder for attack and apparently leave all other tissues untouched. So any straightforward theory for the mutational origin of cancers seemed untenable. In fact, worse was to come.

Following the discovery that repeated applications of tar would regularly produce skin cancer in rabbits and mice, a major effort was launched to identify the active components of tar that were responsible. The thought was that if these could be identified it would be a short step to finding out how they made cells cancerous. The first carcinogens to be purified from tar were certain polycyclic aromatic hydrocarbons.[6] As their name implies, these are compounds of hydrogen and carbon arranged in multiple, unsaturated (or aromatic) rings. The simplest compound, with one ring, is benzene, but as more rings are added more and more arrangements are possible (Figure 5-2). As a group they are widely spread in nature because they are produced from heating almost any organic matter—either quickly when anything is burnt, or slowly over millions of years in warm deposits of oil and coal.[7] The first two pure carcinogens to be identified were dibenz[a,h]anthracene and benz[a]pyrene (shown in Figure 5-2). Unfortunately, as other members of the group were separated and tested for carcinogenicity, it became all too clear that the

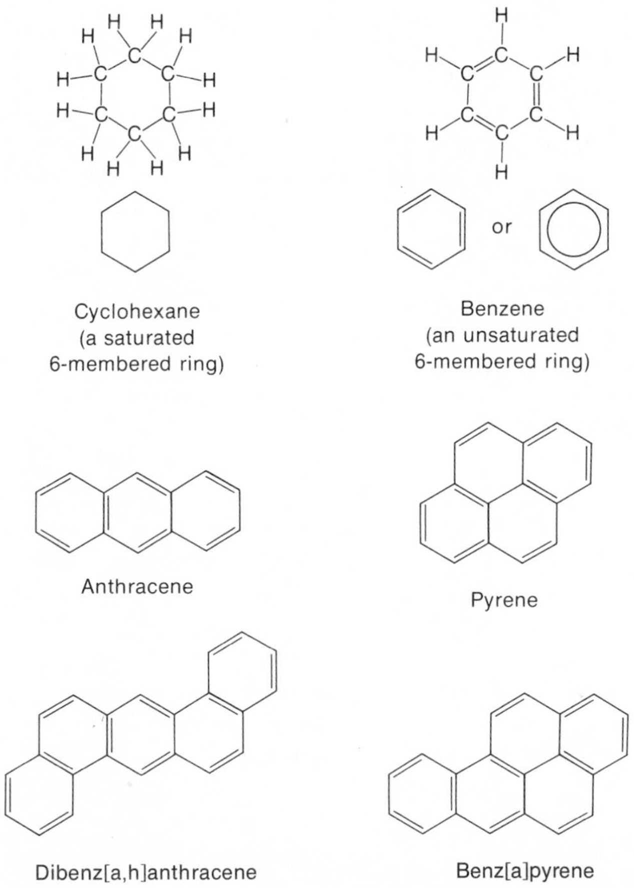

Cyclohexane
(a saturated
6-membered ring)

Benzene
(an unsaturated
6-membered ring)

Anthracene

Pyrene

Dibenz[a,h]anthracene

Benz[a]pyrene

FIGURE 5-2   The carcinogenic polycyclic aromatic hydrocarbons, dibenz-[a,h]anthracene and benz[a]pyrene, are made up of many unsaturated (aromatic) benzene rings. They were among the first chemical carcinogens to be isolated.

exercise was not yielding any profound truth. Admittedly, the carcinogenic members of the group were almost invariably planar and tended to have additional side groups in certain regions of the molecule, whereas highly buckled compounds were not active. But it was not at all clear what this revealed about the mechanism of carcinogenesis. Furthermore, these pure carcinogens proved to be rather unreactive when mixed with various cell components, and—most important—they were not powerful mutagens in any available test system like the fruit fly *Drosophila* or the fungi, yeasts, and bacteria, in which it was easy to measure mutation rates.

Other classes of carcinogen were discovered, and other ways of causing cancer in animals (e.g., X-irradiation), but the basic mechanism of carcinogenesis remained essentially unknown until about 30 years ago. At that time the suggestion was advanced that many of the more inert carcinogens might be dangerous, not in themselves but because they were converted in the body into more reactive compounds,[8] and that a detailed investigation of the metabolism of compounds like benzpyrene should be undertaken.

That idea eventually brought order to much of cancer research, as we shall see later. The other major event was the arrival of molecular biology. In the 1920s and 30s the preoccupation of most biochemists was to determine how cells carry out chemical reactions. Recently, we have started to answer the deeper question of how cells know what to do. This subject, which has been called *molecular genetics,* provides quite a precise picture of the chemical basis of mutation and a fairly clear idea of how mutations are translated into changes in cell behavior. The current dogma is that these recent advances in biology can be turned into a basis for understanding cancer. Therefore the next chapter reviews the origins of molecular genetics and summarizes the current view of how cells store and process information.

MOLECULAR 6 GENETICS, MUTATION, and MUTAGENESIS

The essential property of a cancer cell is that it creates an expanding population of cells like itself. In this sense cancer is an inherited disease. In order to understand it we must therefore first understand something about the chemical basis of heredity.

Since the 1950s, there has been a great outpouring of knowledge in the biological sciences, as there was in physics some 50 years earlier. Because so many of our current ideas about cancer are based on these new discoveries, it is necessary at this juncture to have an interlude in which the reader is introduced to at least the general principles of molecular biology.[1]

The Fundamentals of Molecular Genetics

The branch of science called molecular genetics concerns the area between classical biochemistry and classical genetics—i.e., between the physical details of the chemical reactions carried out by cells in the performance of their various functions and the more abstract study of the way cells inherit from their ancestors the elements (genes) that determine their behavior. For the first half of the 20th century, these two disciplines, biochemistry and genetics, flourished independently. Occasionally some connection was found between them, such as the demonstration that an inherited disease could be due simply to the loss of one particular enzyme. But for the most part the barrier was strictly observed. In the late 1940s two quite separate discoveries opened the way to linking the two disciplines.

At any instant of time, the behavior of a cell is determined entirely by the proteins it has made; most of the chemical reactions going on in the cell are being carried out by protein molecules (enzymes), which have the property of bringing about chemical events that for the most part would not occur spontaneously; and the whole structural organization of the cell is determined primarily by the properties of its various individual structural proteins. The average protein molecule is made up of a hundred or more amino acids, and so contains more than 1000 atoms. Each cell can make several thousand different kinds of protein, and most of these are present in many hundreds or thousands of copies. Because protein molecules were known to be very large and to have a most intricate three-dimensional structure, the problem of determining how any cell could supervise the synthesis of thousands of different proteins, all with exactly the right shape and in the right quantity, was thought to be essentially insoluble.

The great simplification occurred when it was discovered that each species of protein represents a single unbranching chain of amino acids joined in a fixed order, and that the three-dimensional structure of each protein molecule (i.e., the way the chain of amino acids coils up upon itself) is determined automatically by the exact order of the amino acids in this chain. It proved to be possible, for example, to take an enzyme, unravel its chain by altering such conditions as salt concentration and temperature, and then see it reconstitute its original, complex shape and regain its original activity when salt concentration and temperature were returned to their original values (see Figure 6-1). This meant that the cell does not have to mold structure in three dimensions but only place a set of objects (the amino acids) in a correct linear order. Furthermore, because only 20 different kinds of amino acids are used for building proteins, the cell need possess a vocabulary of only 20 different words, plus a few more to mark the end of one protein and the start of the next—words equivalent to "stop," "paragraph" and "chapter"—and some means of controlling how many copies it makes of each protein. In short, the problem of dictating the structure and composition of proteins had become simply that of any conventional written or spoken language.

The second major discovery was made at about the same time—namely that the instructions, which are inherited by each

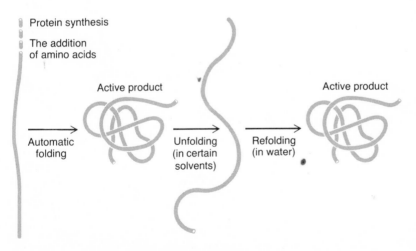

Protein synthesis

The addition of amino acids

Active product

Automatic folding

Unfolding (in certain solvents)

Refolding (in water)

Active product

FIGURE 6-1 The three-dimensional arrangement of each protein chain is determined by the exact sequence of amino acids; the chains automatically fold up so that the most water-soluble amino acids are on the outside and the least soluble on the inside. By making appropriate changes in temperature and solvent it is often possible, for example, to unfold and then refold a protein *in vitro* without permanently altering its properties.

cell and determine the spectrum of proteins in its armory, are
contained in deoxyribonucleic acid (DNA). Nucleic acids are
molecules that, like proteins, consist of unbranching chains of
units or building blocks. The individual units of DNA (the nucleo-
tides or "bases") are four, not 20, and the molecules may contain
millions of units instead of a few thousand. However, there was
obviously no reason why these two languages, one founded on
four letters and the other on 20, should not be linked; after all, we
can communicate in English with the use of either 27 symbols
(the alphabet plus a blank) or 3 symbols (the dot, dash and spacer
of the Morse code).

   Now, it is a very tidy idea that a cell's activity should be determined by two languages: the first language in effect conveys the
cell's inherited instructions to servants (proteins) that use the
second language to execute these instructions. But it did not follow that the idea must be right; and anyway few people at the
time saw the issues in such simple terms. For this reason, the
science of molecular genetics is customarily thought to have
originated a little later with the discovery of the structure of DNA
and the realization of what this structure implied.

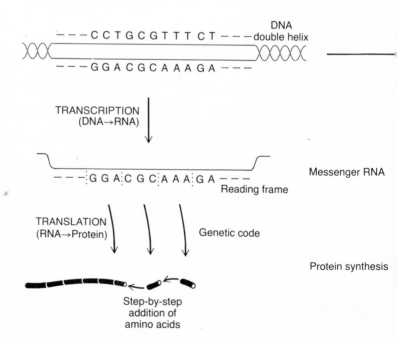

Before any cell divides, it must have duplicated all its information so that it can bequeath a complete set of instructions to each
of its daughter cells. This requirement had always been a problem: in the days when proteins were thought to be the repository
of all the information in a cell, including the genetic information,
it was natural to ask how enzymes are made and, specifically, what
makes the enzymes that synthesize other enzymes. No answer
was forthcoming. But once the genetic information had been
shown to reside in DNA, the problem became that of copying
DNA; how this was done became plain once the structure of DNA
had been discovered. Each molecule turned out to consist of two
separate chains lying side by side that were complementary to
each other in the sense that anyone who knew the sequence of
bases in one chain could write down the sequence in the other.
The foundation of this complementarity is the specific physical
interaction between the four bases found in DNA—adenine,
thymine, guanine, and cytosine: adenine is always placed opposite thymine (and vice versa), and guanine opposite cytosine (Figure 6-2). In order to duplicate such a molecule, it would be neces-

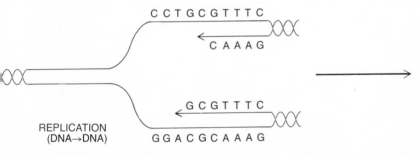

FIGURE 6-2 The replication and expression of genes. The genetic information of the cell
lies in the sequence of bases in its DNA. The bases in the two chains of the DNA double helix
are related to each other by the simple rule of complementarity; cytosine (C) is always opposite guanine (G) or vice versa, and thymine (T) is always opposite adenine (A) or vice versa.

Replication (DNA → DNA). Because the two DNA chains are exactly complementary to each
other, the cell can duplicate its DNA simply by separating the chains and then synthesizing a
new complement to each of them.

Transcription (DNA → RNA). The process of reading the message in the DNA is
accomplished by an enzyme that makes a chain of RNA that is complementary to one of the
DNA chains. Unlike the DNA, this "messenger" RNA is programmed to have a limited lifetime,
and so the cell can change its program of protein synthesis from one moment to the next
without becoming confused by old, outmoded messages.

Translation (RNA → protein). The sequence of bases in the messenger RNA is translated
into amino-acid sequence, the two languages being related by what is known as the genetic
code.

sary only to separate its two chains and then synthesize a new complementary chain alongside each of them. The clinching evidence came in two parts: first the discovery of an enzyme (subsequently named DNA polymerase) that, when given DNA chains, would assemble their complementary chains *in vitro* (i.e., in a mixture in a test tube); second the demonstration that the two chains of a DNA molecule do indeed come apart and go their separate ways when the molecule is duplicated.

These discoveries all occurred in the first dozen years after World War II and have set off a cascade of subsidiary discoveries. The pathway by which the exact sequence of bases in a stretch of DNA is translated into the sequence of amino acids in a protein is now understood in everything but the finer details; this understanding has been achieved by deciphering the *genetic code* and identifying the various *dramatis personae* participating in the act of translation (amounting to roughly one hundred different structural and enzyme proteins plus various smaller molecules). In addition, we now know something about the way these processes are regulated so that a cell can make just the right quantity of each protein, as the need arises.

The primary function of DNA is to dictate the sequence of amino acids in proteins. Using four different bases, the cell must be able to "code for," or specify, the 20 different amino acids plus some form of punctuation. In fact its vocabulary (the *genetic code*) has been shown to consist of the 64 possible three-letter words that can be built out of a four-letter alphabet. Of the 64 words, three are punctuation signals (equivalent to the use of "stop" in a telegram). The remaining 61 words, one of which is a special word for starting proteins, are distributed among the 20 amino acids (i.e., some amino acids are coded by more than one word). No spacers are used, and so in order to get the right message the sequence has to be read in the correct *frame*. Between adjacent regions coding for separate proteins (i.e., between adjacent *genes*) there is always a stretch of DNA, bounded by one or more stop signs and the next start sign. These stretches are not translated but are used for purposes of control (see below). Interestingly, the code is exactly the same for all forms of life, suggesting perhaps that it evolved only once, or that it is the best of all possible codes.

One of the two chains of each DNA molecule contains the message and is identifiable because it also contains appropriate combinations of start and stop signs; the other, complementary chain normally does not contribute to coding (indeed, by definition it does not contain any additional information). The actual process of translating DNA base sequence into protein amino-acid sequence starts with the synthesis of a molecule of a slightly different kind of nucleic acid, not DNA but RNA (ribonucleic acid)—which is complementary to what has been called the "sense" chain of the DNA molecule and extends for the length of the gene. This "messenger" molecule is then translated into amino-acid sequence by a complicated array of enzymatic and structural proteins plus other smaller molecules, in an elaborate sequence of steps that need not concern us here. The important feature of the whole process is that messenger molecules are unstable: thus a cell continues to synthesize each variety of protein only as long as it continues to synthesize the corresponding messenger. It can therefore control its pattern of activities by controlling which messengers are made (i.e., which genes are expressed and which are repressed).

Gene expression is controlled by special proteins whose function is to interact physically with the controlling regions of DNA next to the genes and prevent (or, for some genes, stimulate) messenger synthesis. These repressor proteins are, of course, themselves the product of other genes whose function can be similarly controlled. The operation of a repressor gene is diagrammed in Figure 6-3.

The expression of each gene can therefore be made part of a vast set of interlinked circuits, so that the whole system of genetic instructions becomes rather like the index to an encyclopedia. For example, it is possible to build into the system commands equivalent to saying, "If you know all about molecular biology, skip Chapter 6; if not, you should read the whole of Chapter 6 before proceeding to Chapter 7." Given such regulatory circuits, cells can readily arrange to have two alternate stable states. For example, if Chapter X includes an instruction not to read Chapter Y, and Chapter Y includes an instruction not to read Chapter X, then cells will be enacting either the X program or the Y, but never a mixture of the two. This would therefore constitute a simple form of *differentiation*, and disturbance of such alternate stable states could be part of the process of carcinogenesis.

Most of the preceding information was gained from studying the molecular genetics of bacteria. Multicellular animals are made up of many completely different kinds of cell, all ultimately derived from a single cell (the fertilized egg), and so they have had to develop still more elaborate forms of control. For example,

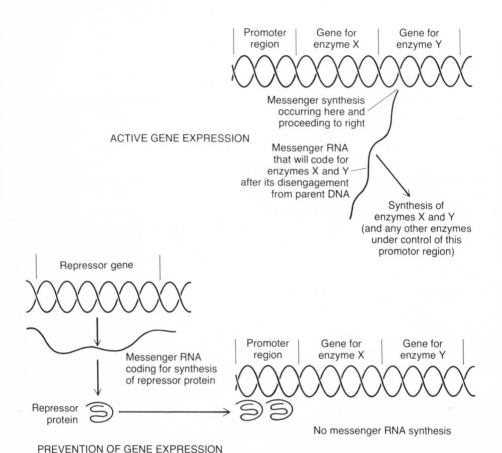

ACTIVE GENE EXPRESSION

PREVENTION OF GENE EXPRESSION

FIGURE 6-3   Gene expression and its prevention. Gene expression is controlled in various ways. In the simplest, shown at bottom, a special "repressor" gene is transcribed into a messenger RNA that codes for the production of a repressor protein. This protein then specifically blocks transcription of one or more genes (shown here as genes for enzyme X and enzyme Y) by binding to the promoter region immediately adjacent to those genes. This prevents the messenger-RNA-synthesizing enzyme from making a message off those genes.

there must be many human genes that are normally expressed only during development of the embryo, and are not meant to be active at any time in adult life. One of the additional methods of genetic censorship used in higher cells is to put several such genes next to each other and then physically compact them together so that they become sequestered and completely inaccessible for messenger synthesis; one such example is the inactivation of X chromosomes which was discussed in an earlier chapter. Very recently, however, two completely unexpected discoveries have been made about the organization of genes in higher cells.

The first discovery concerns the actual structure of the gene. In bacteria, the DNA of each gene consists simply of the sequence of bases that code for some particular protein, plus a short region that determines when the gene is used; in other words, each gene can be likened to a chapter, preceded by a short preface specifying when the chapter should be read. However, it now turns out that the genes of higher cells have a more complex structure because they can contain, actually within the coding sequence, long stretches of DNA that are bypassed during translation (i.e., are not decoded). The function of these strange insertions is still a matter of debate. Understandably, their discovery has left everyone feeling a little discomfited. It is as if we had just graduated to reading more sophisticated textbooks and, on opening the first few, had found that almost every chapter contained several pages which seem to be signifying nothing.

The other discovery is of a somewhat similar kind. Given the very large amounts of information in the DNA of a higher cell (in mammals, a text equal in length to about 20 sets of the *Encyclopedia Britannica*), it was natural to think that the great diversity of function of the different cells of the body was achieved simply by the cells' reading different sections of a huge unchanging textbook—that is, unchanging, except for any chance mutations that might have occurred during the creation of the whole animal from one fertilized egg. It now turns out that the text is not unchanging, but can vary—partly as the result of a predetermined set of rearrangements of fairly long sections of the text, and partly as the result of a high rate of random single-base changes (mutations) confined to certain localized regions of the text. These changes were discovered in the genes that code for antibodies; indeed, this is apparently the way the body manages to code for millions of different kinds of antibody without having to set aside millions of genes for that one task.

The two discoveries force us to accept the idea that in higher cells the readers of the text are fairly versatile and can skip from one section to another (no doubt in a programmed manner) and that the text itself is also somewhat variable (again, in a predetermined way). What effect these ideas will eventually have on our understanding of cancer or on our search for a cure remains to be seen; at the very least, this gives us two more processes that are concerned with the stability (or rather, lack of stability) of the properties of each cell, and either of them could be involved in the chain of events that creates cancer cells.

Mutation

Because each chain of a DNA molecule is faithfully copied when the molecule is duplicated, any change that has occurred in the sequence of bases will thenceforth be handed down from one generation to the next. Such heritable changes are called *mutations*.[?] Let us begin by considering a mutation that occurs simply because at the time of DNA duplication a wrong base is put into one of the new chains. As a result, one of the daughter molecules will have a non-matching pair, and when this region comes to be duplicated again, in the next generation, the mutation will become fixed in one of the granddaughter molecules (Figure 6-4). As it happens, such spontaneous *single-base* changes are exceedingly rare, arising at a frequency of less than one mistake for every 100,000,000 bases copied. This is partly because DNA polymerases are very precise and partly because there seems to be a system of "quality control" operating during the duplication of DNA that monitors all newly made DNA for non-matching pairs and makes corrections wherever necessary.

When one base is changed into another, the effect is much like that of a typographical error—usually negligible, but occasionally devastating. At most positions in the average protein it makes little difference which amino acid is present. Trouble comes only when a significant change occurs in an important part of the molecule (e.g., the active, catalytic site of an enzyme), or when it converts one of the 61 coding triplets into one of the 3 "stop" signs so that the distal end of the gene is not translated and a truncated—and thus inactive—protein is produced.

The result of producing an inactive or altered protein depends on its function. Each of our cells has two copies of nearly every gene (a maternal copy and a paternal one); additionally, most gene products are synthesized in larger quantities than necessary. This means that a mutational defect in just one of the two gene copies may well not lead to disease, because the remaining, normal copy of the gene will synthesize enough normal protein for the needs of the cell. Mutations in such genes are called *recessive*, because they produce disease only when both maternal and pat-

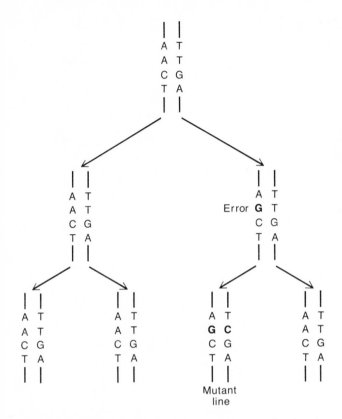

FIGURE 6-4   Mutation due to an error in DNA replication. Any error made during DNA replication will, if uncorrected, become fixed at the next round of replication and give rise to a permanently mutated line. In this diagram we see the result of putting a guanine (G) into the new DNA chain opposite a thymine (T) in the old chain—i.e., into the place that should properly have received an adenine (A); when this region comes to be replicated again, a cytosine (C) will be put opposite that guanine and a mutant line will have been created, in which there is a G-C base pair in place of an A-T pair.

ernal genes are mutant (Figure 6-5a). For example, a mutation in the gene for hemoglobin can lead to a change in one of the amino acids in hemoglobin and this can markedly alter the molecule's physical properties, but overt disease occurs only when both hemoglobin genes contain mutations; and that is why sickle cell anemia, as it is called, is a recessive trait.

For some genes, however, alternation of either of the two copies is sufficient to produce an effect. Thus, any mutation that renders

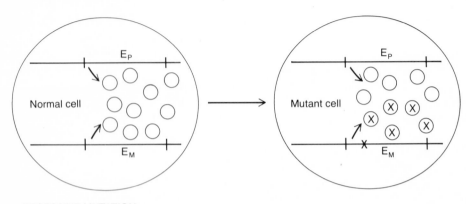

a RECESSIVE MUTATION

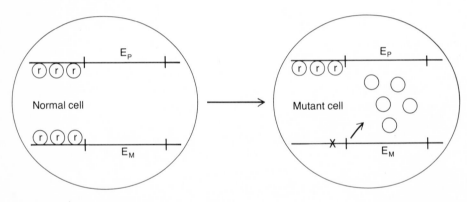

b DOMINANT MUTATION

FIGURE 6-5   Vertebrate cells have two copies of most genes (the maternal and paternal copies), and the effect of any mutation will depend on the type of gene affected.

(a) *Recessive mutation.* If one of the genes for some enzyme, E, contains a mutation (X), the cell will synthesize a mixture of active and inactive enzyme molecules. However, if the enzyme is being made in greater quantity than absolutely necessary for the normal operation of the cell, this mutation in just one of the two genes will not cause any gross abnormality. Such a mutation is therefore called *recessive,* because it becomes manifest only when the other gene copy also is mutated.

(b) *Dominant mutation.* If the gene for a certain enzyme, E, is normally repressed by the binding of repressor protein molecules (r) to its neighboring promoter region, a mutation X in this promoter region can release the gene from this repression. As the result of such a mutation, the gene next to the mutated promoter region will be expressed, and the cell will now acquire a gene product that normally would not be present. Such a mutation is therefore called *dominant* because it is manifest when either maternal or paternal DNA is mutant.

a repressed gene insusceptible to repression will allow the gene to become active, and the cell will therefore acquire a gene product that it otherwise would not contain. Mutations of this kind are called *dominant,* because they produce an effect when either the maternal or the paternal gene is mutant (Figure 6-5b). For example, the commonest cause of human dwarfism is due to a dominant mutation that makes all the long bones of the body stop growing prematurely; the molecular basis of this disease is not known but it is presumably the result of some defect in the interplay of genes that normally occurs in development.

Some very complicated regulatory circuits have been discovered that determine the precise sequence of events in the growth and development of even such simple organisms as bacteria and viruses. But even the most complicated developmental programs prove to be made up simply of sets of coding and regulatory sequences in DNA that interact with each other in various ways. Although we do not know the gene products affected in most genetic diseases of man, there is good reason to think that any change inherited by all the descendants of a cell (and this includes cancer) must be due in some way to a change in the dialogue between nucleic acids and proteins.

Of the various classes of mutation, the simplest is where one base has been changed. A more extensive type of alteration is the removal of a few bases, or the addition of some extra ones. It is not clear what sequence of events can cause this to occur spontaneously, but when it happens within a region of DNA that is coding for a protein and the change in bases is not a multiple of three, the whole reading frame of the gene is of course altered and the resulting protein consists partly of a nonsensical sequence of amino acids. Therefore it is not surprising that—unlike changes in a single base, which are often undetectable—such *frame-shift* mutations almost invariably destroy the function of the gene in which they occur.

Sometimes, much longer sequences of DNA (containing several genes) can be deleted, inverted, or moved from one region to another. Indeed, these rearrangements sometimes occur on such a large scale that they are visible under the microscope. In organisms that are more complicated than bacteria and need a very large amount of DNA with which to conduct their affairs, the DNA tends to be divided up into several packages (chromosomes). Man, for example, has 23 pairs of chromosomes (one member of each pair coming from the mother and the other from the father). Recently methods have been developed for distinguishing microscopically each of the 23, so that any large scale chromosomal rearrangement can now be identified quite precisely.

A good example of a rearrangement causing disease is the shift of a piece of one chromosome-22 to the end of a chromosome-9; this rare change, which will be discussed again on page 140, appears to be the prelude to one form of leukemia. Such rearrangements produce their effects because neighboring parts of a chromosome tend to influence each other's activity. An extreme example is provided by a female's two X chromosomes, one of which is normally rendered totally inactive because it is relegated to one side of the nucleus; when part of some other chromosome becomes translocated into this X chromosome, it is effectively lost because it too becomes inactivated. Indeed it seems likely that, in general, the effects of rearrangement are due either to the repression of genes that should be active, or to the activation of genes that should be inactive.

The three classes of mutation—single-base change, frame shift, and large-scale rearrangement—are illustrated, with English sentences, in Figure 6-6.

All such rearrangements (and perhaps even the small additions or subtractions of bases that cause frame-shift mutations within

(1) Limited changes
Correct message: THE NUN SAW OUR CAT EAT THE RAT
  Single-base change converting one base to another
    Mis-sense
    THE SUN SAW OUR CAT EAT THE RAT
    Nonsense
    THE NSN SAW OUR CAT EAT THE RAT
  Frame-shift changes, as a result of adding or subtracting one base
    THE NUN SAS WOU RCA TEA TTH ERA T

(2) Large-scale changes
Correct message: IF THEY FIND THE NEXT TWO CHAPTERS TOO ABSTRUSE, THEY SHOULD SKIP THEM AND PROCEED STRAIGHT TO CHAPTER NINE.
  Deletion
  IF THEY FIND THE NEXT TWO CHAPTERS TOO ABSTRUSE, THEY SHOULD SKIP CHAPTER NINE.
  Rearrangement
  IF THEY FIND CHAPTER NINE TOO ABSTRUSE, THEY SHOULD SKIP THEM AND PROCEED STRAIGHT TO THE NEXT TWO CHAPTERS.

FIGURE 6-6   Unlike the genetic code (consisting of three-letter words only) our language has words of varying length, but it can be used to illustrate the effects of the main classes of mutation.

single genes) may originate as errors during the process called recombination. Like the two chains of a single DNA molecule which have a direct physical interaction with each other, any two identical or almost identical DNA molecules can interact and exchange homologous segments. The actual biochemistry of this process of *recombination* seems to be very complicated, but the end result is simply that when one of a cell's two copies of a gene undergoes mutation there is a chance that the mutated and un-mutated copies will exchange places at some time or other in the family tree descending from that cell. In this way, new combinations of the many versions (*mutants*) of different genes are continually being created. As a result, natural selection can test the fitness of any new version of a gene not only in its original environment (i.e., with whatever versions of other genes happened to be present on the chromosome at the time it arose) but also when it is combined with other variant forms.

For most multicellular animals, this process of recombination is of course mainly important to the *germ line* (the cells that give rise to sperm and egg) because these are the only cells that can pass mutations on to future generations. So it is not surprising to find that the process of recombination is particularly active during the special cell divisions that immediately precede the formation of egg and sperm. However, recombination can also occasionally occur in cells that are not members of the germ line (i.e., the cells in the rest of the body, which are called the *somatic* cells), and this recombination may be an important factor in the genesis of cancer (see p. 95).

Even the most casual survey shows that mutations and rearrangements are not occurring completely at random; the mutation rate is at least 100 times higher in some human genes than in others, and some rearrangements are much commoner than others. In bacteria and viruses, where genetic analysis can be pursued to the level of the individual bases in a gene, it turns out that a single base out of the hundreds or thousands in a gene may be the site of most of the spontaneous mutations occurring in that gene. Such local regions of instability are called *hot spots*. The pattern of hot spots in any gene is completely different for each of the main classes of mutagenic agent (see the next section), indicating probably that minor differences in the way each section of DNA is coiled and packaged in the cell determine exactly how accessible it is to chemical modification and how likely it is to be erroneously copied or to be misaligned during recombination.

Hot spots may be important in carcinogenesis because they could be one of the factors determining which tissue is most susceptible to which carcinogen.

Chromosomal rearrangements may originate in another way.[3] Recently a novel set of genetic elements have been discovered in bacteria and given the name *insertion sequences*. Each is composed of a stretch of DNA about 1000 bases long. These sequences have the completely unexpected (and as yet unexplained) property of being able to move around from one region of the bacterium's DNA to another or, occasionally, even from one bacterium to the next. Their importance derives from the fact that when they move around they may carry bacterial genes along with them. For example, each time man discovers a new antibiotic, this applies intense selection pressure favoring any rare variant bacteria that have already modified (by chance mutation) one of their enzymes so that the enzyme can break down the antibiotic. If, by chance, the gene for this new enzyme (which now counts as an antibiotic-resistance gene) now happens to become bracketed on either side by insertion sequences it may acquire the insertion sequences' ability to be passed from one bacterium to another. Such complexes of antibiotic resistance genes and insertion sequences are called *resistance transfer factors* and have become one of the major barriers to antibiotic therapy. Elements have been described in plants that bring instability to genes that are near them, but it is not yet known whether insertion sequences will prove to have the same importance in higher forms of life that they seem to have in many bacterial species. This question will be raised again when we consider the behavior of certain tumor viruses.

In this section we have covered very briefly the subject of spontaneous mutation, from changes in a single base in the DNA molecule to the large-scale rearrangement of whole blocks of genes. The rate at which these changes are allowed to occur spontaneously can to some extent be regulated by each species to give it an overall optimum mutation rate.

√ Mutagenesis

When cells are cultivated *in vitro*, they can be pushed into making mistakes during DNA duplication by being fed various unnatural DNA precursors. However, that is a highly artificial situation, and for practical purposes we can regard all mutagenesis as being primarily due to alterations of finished DNA molecules.

Many agents interact with DNA. When they affect the DNA of cells in the germ line, they raise the level of deleterious mutations that has to be borne by future generations; when they affect the DNA in somatic cells of the fetus, they can cause developmental errors that appear as birth defects; and it is thought that when they affect somatic cells in adult life they can cause cancer. It has therefore become an important part of preventive medicine to identify the more potent mutagens in our environment so that they can be either eradicated or at least kept at a safe distance.

Various forms of radiation can damage DNA. The main effect of ultraviolet irradiation is to bind together adjacent bases, particularly when two thymines or two cytosines are next to each other; but because ultraviolet light is not at all penetrating, its effects are confined to our skin and eyes. In contrast, X-irradiation tends to produce breaks in the DNA chains. Because X-rays are highly penetrating, they can affect any cell in the body.

Chemical agents have a wide range of effects. They can remove various side groups from the bases (e.g., nitrous acid removes the amino group from cytosine), or produce cross-links between the two chains of a DNA molecule, or add new chemical groups to the DNA bases (e.g., ethylmethanesulfonate can add methyl groups on to guanine), or even link themselves on to the DNA (e.g., the *diagram* carcinogen benzpyrene becomes linked to guanine). These different alterations can all be observed directly in DNA extracted from cells immediately after they have been irradiated or treated with chemical mutagens, and some of the changes are illustrated in Figure 6-7.

Using certain convenient genes, one can measure the resulting mutation rates. Such comparisons show that far more alterations occur per gene-length stretch of DNA than do final mutations per gene; in other words, only a very small minority of the alterations ever lead to mutation. The reason is that most cells can, to some extent, repair any damaged stretch of DNA.

Nearly everything known about DNA repair has come from experiments with bacteria. These studies have shown that a cell can use a number of different processes to restore a damaged section of DNA. For example the common lesion produced by ultraviolet light, namely the abnormal joining of two adjacent thymines, can be eliminated in at least three different ways. In the neatest of the three, the cell employs a special enzyme that,

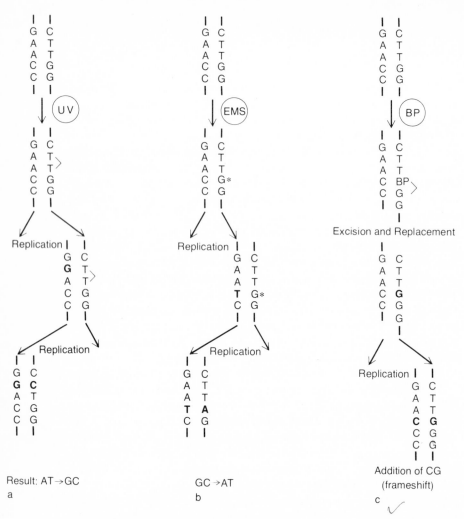

FIGURE 6-7   Different forms of mutagenesis.

(a) *Mutagenesis by ultraviolet light (UV)*. Ultraviolet light is mutagenic because it links adjacent thymines in DNA. Normally these lesions are quickly excised and replaced with unlinked thymines. But if this region of the molecule is replicated before the repair has been made, the new strand may be given an incorrect base opposite one or both of the thymines because the linked thymines are not recognizable as such, and the cell therefore has no way of knowing what the base sequence should be at that point.

(b) *Mutagenesis by ethylmethane sulfonate (EMS)*. EMS can react directly with DNA guanine. The resulting altered guanine (O_6-methyl guanine) tends to be mistaken for adenine when the DNA is subsequently replicated. EMS therefore causes the change of a G-C base pair into an A-T pair.

(c) *Mutagenesis by benzpyrene (BP)*. A carcinogen like BP is mutagenic because when it enters the body it undergoes certain chemical changes and then becomes aligned in the DNA molecule as if it were one of the bases. In this position, it can become bound to neighboring guanines. During the excision and replacement of these BP-guanine complexes, frame-shift mutations are apt to occur.

using the energy of blue light, can simply break the abnormal bonds holding the thymines together and thereby restore the DNA to its original state; this form of repair is called photoreactivation and can be observed not only in bacteria but also in cultured animal cells and even in the skin of an intact animal. In a second repair process, a battery of several gene products between them manage to locate the thymine dimers, cut the DNA chain nearby, excise a region of perhaps about 30 bases, and then re-synthesize a new stretch to replace the old, using the undamaged DNA strand as a template; this process is observed also in higher cells and is important because it too is apparently an error-free way of repairing ultraviolet lesions. In both of these methods the enzymes used are present in cells at all times. In the third process, some of the enzymes employed are formed only when the need arises (e.g., after heavy irradiation); this process produces a lot of errors and is responsible for most of the mutations that follow ultraviolet irradiation. The sensitivity of a population of bacteria to ultraviolet light (i.e., the extent to which they are killed or mutated by a given dose) is determined by the exact balance between these processes of repair, which in turn is affected by how fast the bacteria are multiplying. As one might expect, cells that have a lot of time in which to repair their DNA before being required to duplicate it are much more successful than those with little time to spare. This, incidentally, may be one of the reasons why cancers tend to arise mostly within populations of cells that are multiplying rapidly.

Most chemical mutagens can produce several different classes of lesion in DNA, each of which can probably be handled in a variety of ways. Some of the methods of repair may be the same as those used for ultraviolet lesions, but no doubt there are others still to be discovered. Fortunately most cells appear to react in much the same way to any given mutagen, thus enabling us usually to get a reasonable idea of any new compound's mutagenicity for man by studying its mutagenicity for bacteria; such tests are described in the next chapter.

Any biological process may be rendered partly or completely defective as a result of mutation, and the various methods of DNA repair are no exception. Most of what we know about the different repair processes used by bacteria has come from studying bacterial mutants that have lost the use of one or another process. For example, it turns out that several different proteins must be cooperating in carrying out the error-free excision of ultraviolet lesions (the second process described above) because mutation in any one of several genes will completely block that means of repair and force the bacterium to rely on the other repair processes. Interestingly, a set of completely analogous mutations have been observed in man that give rise to a rare inherited disease, xeroderma pigmentosum, characterized by an increased sensitivity to sunburn plus an increased incidence of skin cancer.

The discovery of the various forms of DNA repair has added a large number of extra components to the list of cell ingredients known to be concerned with the manufacture and handling of what are called the cell's *informational macromolecules* (i.e., the various molecules of nucleic acid). In the most thoroughly studied organism, the bacterium *E. coli*, about 200 distinct species of molecule have been observed, and no doubt many more await detection. This interlocking system of checks and balances may break down at a number of points. And, as in other arenas of life, when things go wrong they can go quickly from bad to worse; for example, any mutation affecting one of the genes whose products monitor for errors made during DNA duplication would tend to raise the mutation rate; this could then produce additional defects and a further increase in mutation rate, and so on. In fact, effects exactly like this have been observed in bacteria as the result of changes in the enzymes concerned with DNA and protein synthesis. Of course, unicellular creatures such as bacteria are not at much risk from any drop in precision, simply because in most situations survival of the fittest means survival of the most precise; in other words, any population of bacteria will automatically tend to cleanse itself of mutants of this class. The same may not, however, be true for long-lived multicellular animals. Indeed, one theory of aging is that our cells accumulate imprecision at a constantly increasing rate as we grow older, because they are not being subjected to any selection pressure in favor of precision.[4] This brings us directly to the role of mutation in the development of cancer, which is discussed in the next chapter.

EXPERIMENTAL CANCER RESEARCH (1): CHEMICAL CARCINOGENS, RADIATION, and VIRUSES

Much of our knowledge of human cancer has derived from epidemiological studies of the kind described in Chapter 4. One approach to a more detailed analysis of the causal processes has been to develop experimental cancers in animals. Another way has been to study the action of known carcinogens upon simple organisms like bacteria. Out of this has come a simple way of testing various agents for their probable carcinogenicity.

It is roughly half a century since ways were found of producing cancers in animals, and by now there is a vast body of information describing the results of administering different agents by different routes and in various combinations to various species. Cancer can be produced by painting substances on to the skin, by feeding, or by injection, and the resulting cancers may develop locally where the carcinogen was applied, or at some remote site. One purpose of all this work has been to determine which agents are the most potent carcinogens and therefore most likely to be dangerous to humans; another, to develop experimental cancers on which to test new forms of treatment. But the primary incentive has been the belief that, by studying the various permutations of carcinogen, dose, duration of treatment, route of administration, species and age of host and so on, someone might discover some fundamental illuminating principle common to all forms of carcinogenesis and then somehow be able to convert this knowledge into a cure for cancer or at least a strategy for preventing it.

A few underlying principles have emerged. For example, so many carcinogens have proved to be powerful mutagens that it seems almost certain that most forms of cancer are due, at least in part, to changes in DNA. But little or nothing is known about the functions of the genes that must be mutated, and there are enough oddities about the whole process of carcinogenesis to suggest that it is not a matter simply of piling one mutation upon another until the requisite number of genes are inactivated but probably involves something else as well. Despite our great ignorance about the basic biology of cancer, the study of carcinogens has recently been made much easier by the application of knowledge and techniques derived from bacterial molecular genetics.

Chemical Carcinogenesis

The conspicuous feature of most forms of carcinogenesis is the long period that elapses between initial application of the carcinogen and the time the first cancers appear. For example, it is necessary to apply coal tar repeatedly to a mouse's skin for several months before any cancers are detectable; similarly, most people do not incur much risk of getting lung cancer until they have smoked for 10 to 20 years. Clearly, we cannot claim to know what turns a cell into a cancer cell until we understand why the time course of carcinogenesis is almost always so extraordinarily long.

Following the discovery that skin cancer could be produced by coal tar, attempts were made to purify the active ingredients responsible. When tar proved to contain many different active components—some more carcinogenic than others and some more irritant than carcinogenic—people began testing various combinations of agents in various sequences; in particular they wanted to find out if the toxic, irritant property of many carcinogens was essential to their action. Out of all this work with coal tar derivatives (and, later, with many other carcinogenic chemicals) an important and unexpected complication came to be recognized. Although it is often possible to produce cancer in an animal by prolonged treatment with a single species of purified carcinogen, in certain situations the process of carcinogenesis can be separated into two distinct steps. These have been called *initiation* and *promotion*.[1]

To take an extreme case, cancer can be produced in mice by feeding them on a single occasion a small amount of dimethyl-benzanthracene, DMBA (one of the active ingredients of coal tar), and then later subjecting their skin to prolonged irritation. The resulting cancers are confined to the irritated regions of skin, but they would not have appeared without the initial treatment with DMBA, or if the DMBA had been administered after the skin had been irritated: this shows that both ingredients are necessary—first the DMBA (the *initiator*) and then the irritant (the *promoter*). Furthermore, the results are not substantially altered if a long interval is interposed between initiation and promotion. Therefore the initiator is producing a permanent, irreversible change in a certain proportion of cells throughout the body, and subsequently the promoter somehow provokes the expression of this change (Figure 7-1).[2]

In the last few years more and more evidence has been accumulating to suggest that initiation is nothing other than mutation. Though admittedly circumstantial, it is very persuasive. Thus, the most powerful initiators prove to be the substances that are the best at binding to DNA (Figure 7-2)[3] and causing mutations in various test systems (see p. 100); they produce changes in DNA either directly, or indirectly after they have undergone certain chemical modifications that occur when they are metabolized in the body (see p. 103). It seems reasonable to

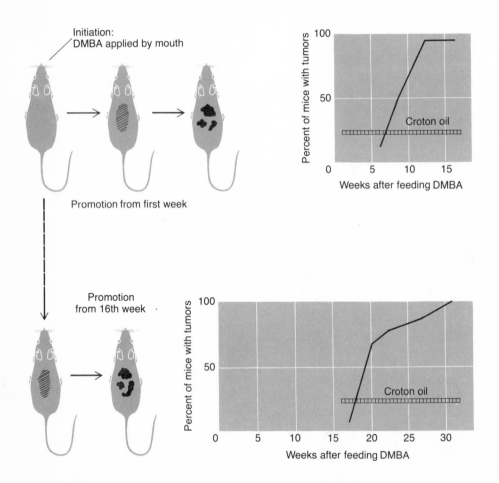

FIGURE 7-1   The separation of carcinogenesis into two stages—initiation and promotion. A group of mice are fed a small amount (25 micrograms) of the carcinogen dimethylbenzanthracene (DMBA) (the "initiator"); this produces widespread irreversible alterations (presumably mutations) in the cells of each mouse. Subsequently, irritation of the skin by painting it twice a week with croton oil (the "promoter") results in the local appearance of tumors. These tumors will appear even if promotion is not started until 16 weeks after the DMBA feeding, but no tumors arise if either DMBA or croton oil is given alone or if the order of the treatments is reversed.

The top graph shows the increase in percentage of mice with tumors, when promotion is started in the first week. The bottom graph shows the increase in percentage of mice with tumors, when promotion is not started until the 16th week. [After R. K. Boutwell, *Prog. Exp. Tumor Res.* **4**, 207–250 (1964). Published by S. Karger AG, Basel.]

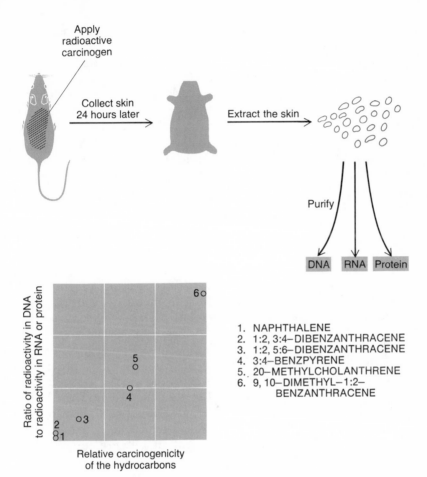

1. NAPHTHALENE
2. 1:2, 3:4–DIBENZANTHRACENE
3. 1:2, 5:6–DIBENZANTHRACENE
4. 3:4–BENZPYRENE
5. 20–METHYLCHOLANTHRENE
6. 9, 10–DIMETHYL–1:2–
         BENZANTHRACENE

FIGURE 7-2   The interaction of initiators with DNA. The carcinogenicity of six different polycyclic aromatic hydrocarbons was shown to be correlated with their ability to bind to cellular DNA when they were painted onto mouse skin. A radioactive derivative of each carcinogen was prepared and applied to the skin of a mouse. After 24 hours, the mice were sacrificed, and the extent to which the radioactivity had become bound to the different components of the cell (e.g., DNA, RNA, and protein) was measured. As the graph at bottom shows, the potency of these compounds as carcinogens is correlated with their propensity to bind to DNA, rather than their propensity to bind to protein. Until this experiment was reported, most people believed that carcinogens acted by modifying proteins (e.g., by affecting repressors and thereby affecting gene expression). [Data after P. Brookes and P. D. Lawley, *Nature* **202,** 781–784 (1964).]

assume that the first step in carcinogenesis would be the production of mutations, because this conforms to the one thing we do know about the cancer cell—namely, that in building up an expanding population of abnormal cells it must be passing on its cancerous characteristics to its descendants, and so these characteristics must in a sense be inheritable from one cell generation to the next.

The nature of promotion is still very obscure, but we get some hints if we consider what substances can act as promoters. For the production of skin cancers in mice the most commonly used promoting agent is croton oil (a blistering agent and purgative extracted from the seeds of an Indian tree); when rubbed on the skin, it produces a local reddening and thickening and temporarily increases the rate of cell proliferation.[4] In rabbits, actual physical wounding will bring on skin tumors initiated with coal tar.[5] For the production of cancer in internal organs, certain special methods of promotion have been found: for example, partial excision of the liver forces the remaining liver cells to multiply and compensate for the loss, and this will promote liver cancer in mice that have been fed an initiating agent; much the same kind of effect has been demonstrated for the thyroid[6] and ovary,[7] where excessive cell multiplication can be provoked by appropriate hormones; similarly, leukemia can be brought on in X-irradiated rats by repeatedly bleeding them so that the cells in their bone marrow have to increase their extent or rate of multiplication.[8]

All these procedures have in common the one feature that they are provoking increased cell multiplication. What remains now is for us to guess why such provoked multiplication should be dangerous to a tissue like skin or marrow, where the cells are multiplying the whole time even in the absence of an artificial stimulus. In fact, no very plausible explanation has emerged, but two possibilities are worth describing if only to illustrate how little we really know about the process of carcinogenesis.

(1) The first is a conventional genetic explanation. Recall that, except for the genes contained in the sex chromosomes (see p. 18), every cell has two copies of each of its genes, one of maternal origin and one paternal, and these are duplicated prior to cell division and then appropriately partitioned (segregated) to its two daughter cells. We might suppose that cancer can occur only when both copies of some particular gene have undergone mutation, i.e., that cancer is "recessive." Such a double event should be rather rare, and we might easily imagine that a much commoner

Genetic theory

way for two mutant copies to occur in the same cell would be by somatic recombination (see p. 83), or alternatively by some mistake at cell division that left one cell with both the copies of a mutated gene (e.g., both paternal genes). Such events are known to occur, albeit very rarely during normal cell multiplication, and promoting agents could conceivably make them more common.

(2) An alternative explanation could be that when cells are forced to multiply quickly they may make mistakes, not in the actual segregation of their DNA, but in the control of expression of this DNA. Each cell in the adult animal is expressing only a small minority of its genes; for example, all our cells have the gene for insulin, but only certain cells in the pancreas are pro-grammed to express that gene. Every one of the unexpressed genes in a cell has been switched off (repressed) by one of the cell's ancestors, at some stage in the development of the embryo; in-deed, the whole program of embryonic development is really a carefully controlled sequence of decisions concerning which genes each cell should be expressing at each stage in develop-ment? These decisions are thought to be perpetuated by the syn-thesis of certain special proteins, that are the product of one set of genes and block or enhance the expression of certain other genes. When any cell is treated with a mutagen, most of the resulting mutations will naturally occur in genes that are repressed and therefore silent, simply because in any cell the silent genes greatly outnumber those that are being expressed. If an animal has been exposed to a mutagen, and some subsequent treatment is applied that tends to activate the repressed silent genes, then in the course of time more and more mutated genes will be revealed; and that may be what promoters are doing. This is an example of what would be called an *epigenetic* explanation, because it attrib-utes promotion solely to alterations in the pattern of gene expres-sion rather than any alteration in DNA base sequence.

Those are just two of the numerous possible explanations of promotion. Many people would say that the problem is entirely artificial because most known chemical carcinogens are complete in themselves and can apparently function both as initiators and as promoters. But the distinction between the early and late steps in carcinogenesis is surely worth making if only to remind us that we really have no idea what is going on during the long interval that usually elapses between the initial stimulus and the final appearance of a cancer. An added practical consideration is that the presence of such long intervals tells us we may sometimes

[margin note:] Epigenetic theory

have to delve far into the past to find the stimulus that started the whole process. Two examples will make the point clear. A few years ago it was reported that simply painting the skin of mice with croton oil twice a week for a period of three to six months was producing skin tumors; but it was then learned that the dealer who supplied the mice reared them in wooden cages that had been treated with creosote, and once he stopped this practice the croton oil ceased to produce tumors; in other words, the mice were being initiated long before the experiment had begun.[10] An analogous situation seems to be that of liver cancer in the Chinese in Singapore; the cancer is confined almost entirely to those who spent their childhood actually in China rather than in Singapore itself,[11] as if initiation only occurs in China but promotion can occur in Singapore.

It is possible, however, that some cancers could be totally epigenetic in origin. For example, when one ovary in a mouse is removed and the other is transplanted to the spleen, the normal hormonal communication between ovary and pituitary is interrupted and, as a result, the transplanted ovarian cells undergo excessive multiplication and, in many such mice, proceed to form cancers.[12] It is difficult to see how mutagenesis can have any bearing on the process, and the conventional explanation is that this form of carcinogenesis is strictly epigenetic and due to errors in gene expression. A somewhat similar result has been obtained by transplanting cells of the embryo to the testis;[13] and in this instance additional support for an epigenetic explanation comes from the observation that the resulting cancer cells can be restored to normal behavior by being transplanted into an early developing embryo.[14]

There is another unusual form of carcinogenesis that may also be epigenetic, rather than mutational, in origin. When plastic films are implanted subcutaneously in rodents they give rise to cancers (fibrosarcomas) in the surrounding tissues.[15] The process seems to depend on interrupting the normal communication between cells, because it can be caused by any solid surface (plastic or metal) but does not occur if the film has been broken up into small pieces or contains holes through which the cells can pass extensions of their cytoplasm.[16] Similar cancers occasionally occur in human scar tissue.[17] However, the mechanism underlying such *physical carcinogenesis*, as it is called, seems just as obscure as it was for the examples mentioned in the preceding paragraph.

Although, as we shall see, most known human carcinogens prove to be mutagens, it is important to remember that some of the cancers for which no cause has been discovered may be partly due to agents that are not mutagens but act instead by provoking cell multiplication and errors in gene expression.

Testing for Mutagenicity and Carcinogenicity

Nearly all known chemical carcinogens turn out to be mutagens. Therefore the search for the agents in our environment that cause cancer tends to be regarded as just one aspect of a general search for agents that cause mutation.

When a mutagen affects cells in the germ line (ova, sperm, or their precursors), it produces mutations that will burden future generations. When it affects one of the vast majority of cells in the body that are not part of the line of descent from parent to off-spring (the somatic cells), the resulting *somatic mutations* will be confined to whatever family of cells results from division of the mutant (e.g., any cancer that is produced), but they will not be passed on to future generations. Anyone looking for germ-line mutagens is concerned about the future; anyone looking for car-cinogens is interested in protecting the present generation.

At first sight, it might seem easier to produce mutations of the germ line than to produce cancers. Mutation is the immediate and direct result of damage to DNA, and a cell can become a mutant as a result of a single exposure to a mutagen, whereas most forms of cancer emerge only after prolonged exposure to carcinogens. Nevertheless, historically the discovery that some-thing was a carcinogen nearly always preceded discovery that it was a mutagen. X-rays were discovered in 1895 and seven years later a skin cancer was observed on the hand of a man whose occupation was making and testing X-ray tubes; but 25 years were to elapse before X-irradiation was shown to increase the mutation rate of the fruit-fly *Drosophila*.[18] Similarly, car-cinogenesis by certain industrial chemicals was observed in fac-tory workers in 1902 and was demonstrated in experimental animals in 1915, but it was not until 1941 that mustard gas was shown to be mutagenic, once again in *Drosophila*.[19]

Part of the difficulty in detecting mutagens is due to the fact that germ-line cells are well protected from attack by the envi-ronment. Most highly reactive agents that are capable of interacting directly with DNA *in vitro* are intercepted long before they can reach the germ cells, and for an animal like a mouse or a man the most potent agents for raising the frequency of mutations among offspring are penetrating agents such as X-rays. In contrast, tissues such as skin are more directly exposed to the environment and here the main protection against mutagenesis seems to be that more than one mutation must occur in any skin cell in order to convert it to a cancer cell which would endanger the life of the host.

Another difficulty lies in the question of numbers. When you apply a carcinogen to the skin on the back of a mouse, you are presumably testing millions of cells and will detect the conversion of a single one of them into a cancer cell; further, even though this conversion may require several independent mutations, you can continue applying the carcinogen until the key set of mutations is produced. When, however, you are looking for mutations in the germ line, it is not practical (unless you are working with microorganisms) to embark on any experiment that will require looking at more than a few thousand animals.

Many different tests have been employed at one time or another in the screening of compounds for their mutagenicity or carcinogenicity. One of the problems is that most mutations lead to loss of function, rather than creation of a new function, and so are recessive (and therefore detectable only when both maternal and paternal copies of a gene are affected). The exception is mutation in the X chromosome since only one active copy of this chromosome is present in each cell. Thus the simplest test for mutagenesis in an animal is to look for sex-linked lethal mutations in the X chromosome: this was how the mutagenicity of X-rays and mustard gas was discovered. The time required to carry out such a test depends on how long the animal takes to produce offspring (a few days for *Drosophila*), and the sensitivity of the test depends simply on how many offspring you are prepared to count. Testing a compound for carcinogenicity is much more time-consuming and expensive. Thus, in order to be reasonably sure that a new food additive is safe for human consumption it should first have been fed to animals for most of their lifetime (e.g., to mice for more than a year); further, it should have been tested in several different species, because susceptibility to different carcinogens is known to vary widely. For example, the industrial chemical, 2-naphthylamine, which causes bladder cancer in humans, is a fairly potent carcinogen for dogs and hamsters, but not for rats, mice, or rabbits;[20] similarly the fungal products called aflatoxins, which cause general liver damage in poultry and liver tumors in trout, are carcinogenic for rats (but not mice) and possibly for humans (but not monkeys).[21]

In recent years, however, we have begun to learn what underlies these enormous differences between species in susceptibility to particular carcinogens; as a fortunate by-product of this understanding it has been possible to devise much quicker and cheaper tests for carcinogenicity. The argument was first clearly stated in 1946,[22] and has been amply substantiated since then. It runs as follows. The cells in the body are protected by several barriers against the various noxious chemicals in our environment; perhaps the most important barrier is that the superficial layers of cells in the skin and intestine are being continually discarded; as a result the most highly reactive compounds in our environment interact predominantly with cells that are going to be shed. Therefore some of the most dangerous chemicals are not those that from the outset are chemically reactive, but those that are more stable so that they are absorbed unchanged and then become activated during their metabolism in the body. Thus, the variation of different species in susceptibility to given carcinogens is due not to any fundamental difference in the mutability of their DNA, but simply to minor differences in the way each species metabolizes these carcinogens.

The clearest example of a group of carcinogens that have to be metabolically activated are the polycyclic aromatic hydrocarbons, found in coal tar. In the form in which they naturally occur they do not react chemically with DNA and thus are not potent mutagens. However, when they enter the body they are detoxified in a succession of steps (oxidation, hydrolysis and conjugation with various water-soluble substances like glucuronic acid) and then finally excreted (see Figure 7-3). At some of the intermediate stages of the reaction, they may become highly unstable compounds that are able to act as powerful mutagens because they can readily interact with DNA. Whether an animal is susceptible to this form of carcinogenesis may therefore depend on which of its detoxifying enzymes are the most active— those producing mutagenic intermediates or those that further break down these intermediates. For example, the rate-limiting step producing the active intermediate of the carcinogen 3-methylcholanthrene is carried out by the enzyme arylhydrocarbon hydroxylase; this enzyme is deficient in many strains of mice and

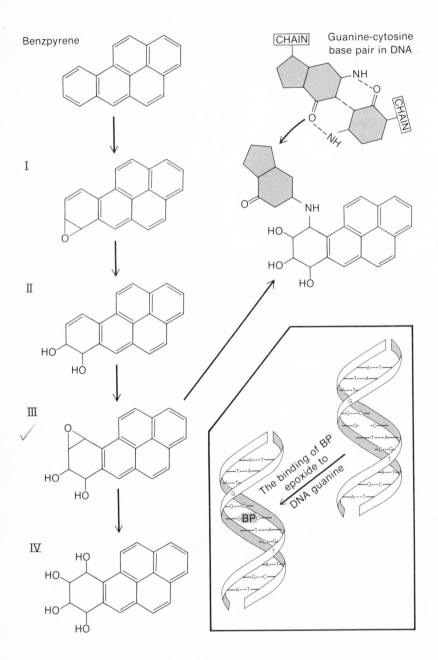

FIGURE 7-3   The detoxification and metabolic activation of benzpyrene. The detoxification of the carcinogen benzpyrene (BP) goes through several steps, as it is made more water-soluble prior to excretion. One of the intermediates in this process (III) is capable of reacting with guanine in DNA (as shown to the right of the diagram). This leads to a massive distortion of the DNA molecule and forces the cell into an error-prone form of DNA repair. Benzpyrene is therefore a mutagen for any cell that has the enzymes that produce this intermediate. [After I. B. Weinstein et al., *Science* **193**, 592–595 (1976).]

although these strains are more sensitive to the immediate toxic effects of many hydrocarbons (reminding us that the primary function of the activating enzymes is detoxification) they are much less susceptible to carcinogenesis by methylcholanthrene than strains that have the enzyme.[23]

In fact the situation is more complicated than this, because these detoxifying enzymes tend to be made by cells only when the need arises (i.e., the enzymes are *inducible*), and many compounds (such as the common sedative phenobarbital) can act as inducers even though they themselves are not potential carcinogens.[24] It is possible therefore to raise or lower an animal's sensitivity to a given carcinogen by prior exposure to substances that are not carcinogens for the tissue being tested; for example, dimethylbenzanthracene will produce mammary cancer in rats, but their susceptibility to this form of carcinogenesis is greatly reduced if they have been treated 24 hours earlier with methylcholanthrene.[25]

It is not yet clear whether people are like mice and vary in their susceptibility to carcinogens through variation in the inducibility of their detoxifying enzymes. Certainly, the level of the enzyme arylhydrocarbon hydroxylase in the placenta is raised to a highly variable extent in women who smoke.[26] Furthermore two studies have reported that the probability of smokers getting lung cancer is related to the amount of this enzyme that can be induced in their lymphocytes.[27] Interestingly, the cells of long-lived animals such as humans and elephants are much less active in converting substances into carcinogens than are the cells of short-lived animals such as rodents.[28]

The discovery of the part played by metabolic activation has had an enormous impact on the techniques for testing compounds for carcinogenicity. As long as powerful carcinogens like dimethylbenzanthracene could not be shown to cause mutations in simple organisms like bacteria, the whole question of carcinogenesis remained shrouded in mystery. When it became apparent that bacteria are insusceptible to many carcinogens simply because they lack the essential activating enzymes,[29] several investigators developed tests in which mammalian enzymes were used in combination with bacteria bearing appropriate genetic markers. The very first tests were unnecessarily laborious but they established the principle.[30] For example, the industrial solvent dimethylnitrosamine was known to be a powerful carcinogen even though it is not a mutagen for bacteria; it could, however, be shown to undergo conversion into a mutagen during its metabolism in mice because test bacteria, temporarily implanted into such mice and subsequently retrieved, were shown to have been mutagenized (Figure 7-4). The bacteria used in this test were a special laboratory strain of *Salmonella typhimurium* bearing a revertible mutation (either a single-base change or a frame shift) in one of the genes for synthesis of the amino acid

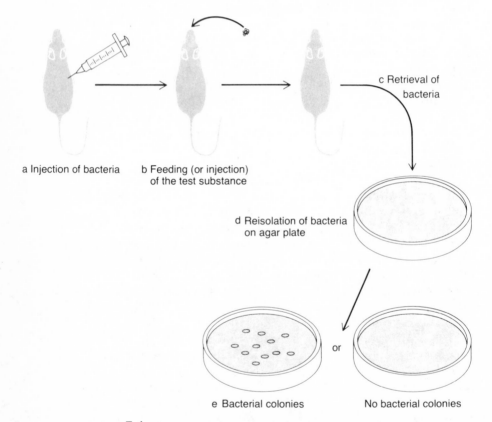

FIGURE 7-4   A test for the formation of mutagens by metabolic activation. (a) The animal is injected with bacteria that have a revertible mutation in the gene for making the amino acid histidine. (b) It is then fed or injected with the substance being tested for mutagenicity. (c) A few hours later the bacteria are retrieved. (d) They are reisolated and spread onto an agar plate that contains every required nutrient except histidine. (e) If the test substance is metabolized in the mouse to yield any compounds that are mutagenic, the bacteria will have undergone mutation and some of them will now be able to grow in the absence of histidine and therefore will form colonies. [After M. G. Garridge et al., *Science* **163**, 689–691 (1969) and *Proc. Soc. Exp. Biol. Med.* **130**, 831–834 (1969).]

histidine; until the mutation is reverted, therefore, these bacteria cannot grow in the absence of added histidine.

Since then, several much simpler methods have been devised that do not require the use of a living animal as an intermediary. The best known test consists of putting the same bacteria on an agar plate containing (1) a nutritional medium that fulfills every requirement for growth except histidine, (2) an extract of liver derived from rats that have been treated with a substance like phenobarbital or methylcholanthrene to induce high levels of the enzymes that activate carcingens, (3) various quantities of the substance that is being tested. If the substance can be converted into a mutagen that produces the appropriate base change or frame shift required to revert the histidine mutation, some of the bacteria will grow and form visible colonies (Figure 7-5).

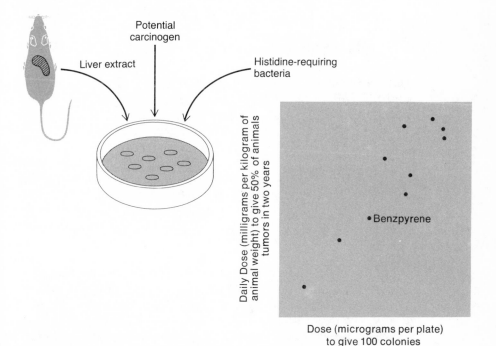

FIGURE 7-5   In this test for the formation of mutagens by metabolic activation, an extract of liver cells is used to provide the activating enzymes, instead of an entire animal. The extract, the potential carcinogen, and the bacteria are all placed on the same agar plate. [After J. McCann et al., *Proc. Natn. Acad. Sci. U.S.A.* **72,** 5135–5139 (1975).

The beauty of a test like this is that it costs about one-thousandth as much as a test using mice, and takes a day or two instead of at least a year. Roughly 90% of known carcinogens prove to be mutagenic to bacteria when activating enzymes are present—about as good a result can be obtained with any one animal species—and more than 90% of substances thought not to be carcinogenic are negative in the test.[31]

Because such microbiological assays are so inexpensive, it has now become practical for the major chemical manufacturers to investigate the potential mutagenicity of all the new compounds they wish to market, before making any major investment to produce them. Anything that comes out positive can then be withheld and tested in animals. The hope therefore is that in future we can avoid inadvertently releasing any really dangerous carcinogens upon the world. Other applications of such tests will be mentioned later.

Radiation Carcinogenesis

Both electromagnetic radiation (e.g., ultraviolet light and X-rays) and particulate radiation (electrons, neutrons, and alpha particles) can damage DNA, cause mutations, and give rise to cancer.[32] In many respects, their action is like that of chemical carcinogens; but it is easier with radiation to study the relationship between mutation rate and dose. For example, it is possible to calculate the exact rate at which natural background radiation produces breaks in each cell's DNA, whereas there is at present no way of determining how efficiently low levels of natural toxic substances such as benzpyrene penetrate the body and are converted into derivatives that can cause mutation.

From what is known about the way cells repair lesions to their DNA, it is clear that there could be several possible relationships between radiation dose and response. Consider the example of mutagenesis of bacteria by ultraviolet light.[33] The main effect of ultraviolet light is to produce bonds between adjacent bases in DNA, giving rise to what are called *dimers*. The number of dimers produced in a cell's DNA is directly proportional to the total dose of ultraviolet light it has received; but once the dimers have been formed, their subsequent effect will depend on whether they are correctly repaired. If the probability of each dimer being incorrectly repaired has a constant value independent of other events in the cell, the number of mutations will also be directly proportional to dose. However, the mechanism that excises dimers and replaces them with normal bases is virtually error free; and so it is only when two dimers happen to be created close to each other on opposite chains of a DNA molecule, and their two regions of repair overlap, that this mechanism can no longer operate and errors will occur; the frequency of such double events will of course be proportional to the square of dose.* An added complication is that bacteria have another mechanism for repairing ultraviolet dimers: this one is induced by radiation and is highly error prone. Judging from what is known about bacteria, therefore, the mutation frequency in animal cells might sometimes increase in direct proportion to dose, or to the square of the dose, and sometimes mutation might occur only when the dose rate is above a certain threshold.

Other forms of radiation tend to break chemical bonds rather than make new ones, and the most easily measured lesions are breaks in the DNA chain. The weaker forms of radiation such as X-rays produce single-chain breaks and these, like ultraviolet dimers, can be repaired by excision followed by the synthesis of a new region using the other, undamaged DNA chain as template; in order for mutation to occur, therefore, two independent events are usually required—one in each chain—so that the mutation rate tends to increase as the square of the dose. The more energetic forms of radiation (e.g., neutrons) commonly break both chains of the molecule, and so interaction with a single neutron can cause mutation; i.e., mutation rate increases in direct proportion to dose. This distinction was demonstrated most clearly by the two atom bombs dropped over Japan. The bomb dropped on Nagasaki produced mostly X-rays and in that city the subsequent incidence of leukemia seems to have been proportional to the square of the dose; in Hiroshima, where the bomb produced a large flux of neutrons, leukemia was proportional directly to dose (Figure 7-6).[34]

By comparison with certain chemicals, most forms of radiation seem to be fairly weak carcinogens. In total, about two hundred cases of leukemia (plus approximately the same number of other

---

*The probability that two events occur is the product of their individual probabilities. For example, the chance of drawing the ace of spades from a deck of cards is one in 52; the chance of drawing it from two successive decks is one in 52^2 (i.e., one in 2704). Similarly, the chance that radiation will produce two lesions in a given region of DNA is the square of the chance that it produces a single lesion and therefore will increase in proportion to the square of the dose of radiation.

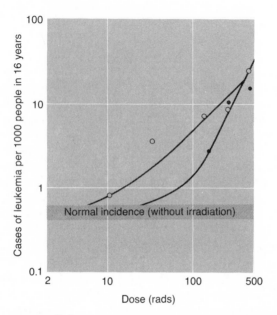

FIGURE 7-6   The incidence of leukemia, within a 16-year period, in Hiroshima and Nagasaki. The incidence produced by the neutrons of the Hiroshima bomb increased in direct proportion to the dose; that produced by the X-rays of the Nagasaki bomb, increased as the square of the dose. Hiroshima incidence, ○ . Nagasaki incidence, ● . [After H. H. Rossi and A. M. Kellerer. *Radiat. Res.* **58,** 131–140 (1974).]

kinds of cancer) were caused by the two atom bomb explosions, and this figure is probably lower than the number of lung cancers arising each year in the two cities as a result of cigarette smoking.

It is easy to exaggerate the long-term hazards of radiation and forget the benefits. For any country with a high rate of tuberculosis (and until recently most Western nations were in this category) the lives saved by mass programs of diagnostic chest X-ray far outnumbered any cancers that might have been caused. Only when we come to less rewarding programs, such as the diagnostic X-irradiation used in screening for breast cancer (see p. 156) do the gains diminish until they are close to the expected losses, and the exact method of calculating losses becomes critical. Precisely the same problem arises when we try to calculate the consequences of exposing a large population, such as a whole nation, to very small doses of a chemical carcinogen. So the exact relation between dose and response is not simply a matter of academic interest.

One last feature of radiation carcinogenesis should be mentioned. As in chemical carcinogenesis, the exact response depends on the form of the radiation and the species of animal. Sometimes the reason for a tissue being affected is obvious; for example, in all species (man included) the ingestion of radium or radioactive strontium tends to produce bone cancers simply because these elements are treated by the body like calcium and are deposited in bone, which they then irradiate by radioactive decay; similarly, radioactive iodine tends to produce cancer of the thyroid. But in any particular species there is no obvious reason why some tissues are selected for carcinogenesis and others are not. In human beings, radiation increases the incidence of myeloid leukemia and cancer of many other sites (e.g., thyroid, skin, and breast); interestingly, although radiologists suffer skin cancer on their hands, the cancers arise only on the backs of their hands, not the palms.[35] In some strains of mice the main response to whole-body irradiation is mammary cancer; in others, it is leukemia (although here there is the complication that the leukemia usually arises in the thymus, which curiously need not itself have been irradiated in order to produce the response);[36] other strains form lung tumors.

Some of the variation in the response of different tissues to chemical carcinogenesis could be attributed to variation in the levels of the enzymes activating the carcinogens. But the exact response to whole-body irradiation with penetrating X-rays is almost as variable from one species to another as the response to chemical carcinogenesis,[37] even though it must be producing lesions in the DNA of every cell. So we are left to conclude that the routes by which cancer cells are created probably differ from one tissue to another. In other words we should not expect to find particular genes, or sets of genes, involved in all forms of carcinogenesis. This is a conclusion that will be reinforced in later sections.

Viral Carcinogenesis

There are many idiosyncrasies in the response of animals to chemical carcinogens and radiation, and it is not clear whether the important steps are genetic or epigenetic. But we do have some idea of what is going on, and believe, for example, that any particular form of chemical carcinogenesis can be explained in terms of fairly simple processes like metabolic activation, errors in DNA repair, and changes in gene expression. The process of viral carcinogenesis is more elusive perhaps because it involves two biological entities, the virus and the host. These usually interact in a very complicated way, and the production of tumors seems to be an almost accidental by-product of the whole process. Before discussing viral carcinogenesis, we must review the kinds of interaction viruses may have with their hosts.[38]

The most conspicuous viruses are those that cause epidemic diseases such as smallpox, measles, influenza, and poliomyelitis. It is now clear, however, that these diseases are not typical of the usual relationship of virus and host but represent unstable situations in which a virus is in the process of adapting to a new host. For example, measles virus produces a lifelong immunity in humans, and so it cannot survive in small communities because it runs out of susceptible hosts;[39] we can deduce therefore that the disease, as we know it, must have arisen in the past thousand years or so because only since then have populations been large enough to sustain it (in fact, it is related to the virus that causes the more chronic disease of canine distemper, and so it may originally have been a disease of dogs). The natural tendency is for viruses to drift towards lower levels of virulence and a more protracted interaction with their host. One example will make this clear. Myxoma virus was introduced into Australia in 1950 and initially caused a rapid fulminating disease in the rabbits, with a mortality of more than 99%; however, the infectious stage of the disease was very short. This meant there was marked survival advantage for variants of the virus that produced a milder and more drawn out disease, because rabbits with a milder disease can be a source of virus for a much longer time than rabbits that die quickly; such variants have now taken over and the mortality of the disease is down to about 25% (Figure 7-7).

At the next level of adaptation of viruses, virulence has declined still further. Take polio virus. In primitive communities each infant is soon infected, but the virus seldom spreads beyond the intestinal tract and so the child becomes a symptomless excreter of virus while it is establishing the immune response that will protect it thereafter against reinfection. When, however, general hygiene is improved, the natural balance between virus and host, that evolved in the course of thousands of years, is suddenly dis-

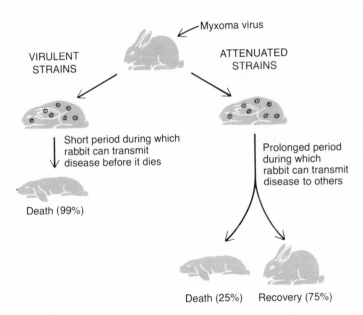

Myxoma virus

VIRULENT
STRAINS

ATTENUATED
STRAINS

Short period during which
rabbit can transmit
disease before it dies

Prolonged period
during which
rabbit can transmit
disease to others

Death (99%)

Death (25%)   Recovery (75%)

FIGURE 7-7   Any strain of virus that quickly kills its host has a lower survival
advantage in nature than less virulent strains, and so there is an almost
inevitable tendency for viruses to acquire a milder, more extended interaction
with their hosts. The first stages of this process are shown particularly clearly by
myxoma virus, which has changed markedly in the last 25 years.

turbed; infection tends to be postponed until after infancy and for
some reason this greatly increases the chance of spread of virus to
the central nervous system. In one sense, therefore, epidemic
paralytic poliomyelitis is a new, man-made disease; indeed, the
first recorded outbreak did not occur until the end of the 19th
century.

The next stage in the adaptation of a virus is to evolve a still
more extended interaction that makes the host a repository and
source of virus for its entire lifetime; this requires a certain
degree of acceptance by the host's immune system. Consider
lymphocytic choriomeningitis (LCM) virus, which is very widespread in mice. Infection normally occurs at birth before the
mouse's immune system is fully effective, and therefore the viral
proteins become accepted by the developing immune system (i.e.,
are classified as "self" rather than "not-self") and this leads to a
permanent state of *tolerance*; there is no immune response and
virtually every cell in the mouse becomes permanently infected
and continually produces small amounts of virus.[40] If, however,

exposure to the virus is postponed until the mouse is an adult, the infection produces a fatal disease of the central nervous system; the disease is apparently due partly to the strong immune response of adult mice because it can be prevented by treating with immunosuppressive drugs.[41] In other words the adult's immune response to this virus seems to be a liability rather than an asset.

The last stage of adaptation is for a virus to become a permanent occupant of all cells, including those of the germ line. This transition is seen in the mammary tumor viruses of mice, some of which are transmitted in the milk (i.e., like LCM virus, infect every mouse soon after it is born) and others are "vertically" transmitted in sperm and ova.[42]

For viruses to persist within their hosts for long periods they must find some way of precisely matching their own replication rate with the multiplication of the cells they are inhabiting. Similar transmissible agents in bacteria have two ways of maintaining a balance with their hosts: either they can remain separate in the bacterial cytoplasm but respond to exactly the same signals that trigger the replication of the bacterial chromosome, and in this state they are called *plasmids*; or they can actually integrate their DNA into the bacterial chromosome so that they are thenceforth carried from one generation to the next just like any other bacterial gene, and in this state they are called *proviruses*. Animal viruses exhibit the same two strategies, plus a few others. Some viruses become integrated into the host's DNA; when the virus nucleic acid happens to be RNA (see p. 75) the process of integration requires that the base sequence first be transcribed into the corresponding DNA sequence; this is what happens, for example, when the cell is infected with mouse mammary tumor virus and Rous sarcoma virus. Others like the herpes group of viruses, which can cause life-long infection in humans (e.g., the cold sores of the lip produced by herpes simplex virus) and seem to be the best candidates for being human tumor viruses, are probably not integrated; rather they appear to persist in the same state as a bacterial plasmid, expressing some of their genes and not others and seldom being packaged into finished virus particles. Others, like LCM virus of mice, continue to multiply slowly so that all cells are producing small amounts of virus the whole time; that is possible, of course, only if the host refrains from producing antibodies against the viral proteins that are being continually produced, and for this to occur the infection must have been established early in life so that the viral proteins are tolerated as if they were host proteins. Others, like human wart virus and the papilloma virus of rabbits, have a variable interaction with cells; they are present in latent form, perhaps as plasmids, in the basal cells of the skin and become converted into infectious particles as soon as the cells start to differentiate. Examples of different interactions between virus and cell are shown in Figure 7-8.

Like the end results of any other evolutionary process, these forms of interaction between virus and host were brought about by a combination of spontaneous mutation and natural selection, operating on both parties but more rapidly on the virus simply because it reproduces faster and is present in greater number. The selection is all the time for a *modus vivendi* that will yield the greatest number of progeny from each of the participants, and it is important to remember that the production of overt disease indicates failure rather than success.

So much for the general properties of viruses and the ways in which they are found to interact with their hosts. When we consider the viruses that can cause tumors in animals,[43] it becomes important to draw a clear distinction between those that produce tumors in natural populations and those that can be made to do so under laboratory conditions. We are interested in the natural tumors of animals because they are potentially models of human disease; if some natural cancers of animals are caused by viruses, so presumably are some human cancers. The viral cancers that can be produced in the laboratory may not be good models of natural disease—indeed, as we shall see, some are plainly laboratory artifacts; but they seem to provide a convenient way of studying the basic biology of the cancer cell. In the remainder of this section we will discuss certain natural cancers of animals and then two forms of artifact—first, the special cancers that can be produced by viruses in the laboratory and, second, the possibility that certain laboratory manipulations may have actually created new tumor viruses *de novo*.

One of the clearest forms of natural viral carcinogenesis is feline leukemia.[44] This is due to a virus, FeLV (feline leukemia virus), that spreads "horizontally" from one cat to another and can be the cause of several distinct diseases. Most infected cats develop a strong antibody response and become immune. But occasionally something seems to go wrong with the response, perhaps because the cells of the immune system are themselves one of the major targets of the virus. Then the cat can suffer either a massive destruction of its immune system (leading to generalized depopulation of the marrow, or a secondary, fatal peritonitis) or a continued uncontrolled proliferation of both

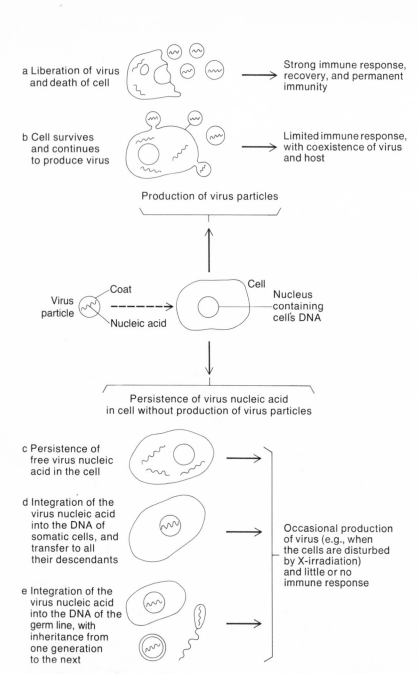

a Liberation of virus and death of cell → Strong immune response, recovery, and permanent immunity

b Cell survives and continues to produce virus → Limited immune response, with coexistence of virus and host

Production of virus particles

Virus particle — Coat — Nucleic acid ------> Cell — Nucleus containing cell's DNA

Persistence of virus nucleic acid in cell without production of virus particles

c Persistence of free virus nucleic acid in the cell →

d Integration of the virus nucleic acid into the DNA of somatic cells, and transfer to all their descendants →

e Integration of the virus nucleic acid into the DNA of the germ line, with inheritance from one generation to the next →

Occasional production of virus (e.g., when the cells are disturbed by X-irradiation) and little or no immune response

FIGURE 7-8   Viruses can interact with cells in many different ways. Some possible results of infection are the following: (a) smallpox and influenza; (b) LCM in mice and possibly the chronic carrier state of hepatitis virus in humans; (c) and (d) the chronic infection with herpes in humans; (e) infection of mice with certain mammary tumor viruses.

virus and responding lymphocytes leading to a disease that is classified as leukemia or lymphosarcoma. It is possible that the leukemia is not due to any direct specific interaction between tumor virus and cell, like the interaction of a cell with a mutagen, but is some nonspecific aberration of the immune response due to the presence of large quantities of virus.

A rather similar disease is seen in mice. Some inbred strains, at about the age of six months, show a high incidence of leukemia associated with massive production of a virus called MLV (murine leukemia virus);[45] the disease can, however, be prevented by greatly restricting the diet (Figure 7-9),[46] and this suggests that the disease may be triggered initially by some slight imbalance between virus production and immune response; incidentally, a similar effect has been reported for limiting diet[47] and for chronic parasitic infection[48] in the case of mouse mammary tumors associated with mammary tumor virus. Recently, some natural isolated colonies of mice have been found which are full of MLV and develop leukemia when captured and kept well fed under laboratory conditions.[49] MLV, like FeLV, belongs to a closely related group called the type-C RNA viruses, that are also found in birds and many different mammals. In many cases, they seem to have evolved a stable relationship with their natural hosts and do not cause any disease under natural conditions. Whether they participate in the genesis of human leukemia is open to argument.

The foregoing cancers all affect mesodermal cells, in particular those of the immune system. However, several natural epithelial tumors of animals are also plainly due to viruses. The best known example is the common human wart. Such viral tumors of the skin are seen in many species and, like the human wart, most of them are benign (i.e., not invasive) and eventually undergo regression due to an immune response to the virus. But a few virus-caused epithelial tumors are not benign. For example, mammary cancer in certain inbred strains of mice is associated with an RNA virus that can be either inherited in the germ line or transmitted in the milk;[50] as mentioned above this cancer too, like murine leukemia, also depends on appropriate dietary factors. (In other species, such as the rat,[51] mammary cancers arise that are not demonstrably associated with any virus.) Although the search for human mammary cancer viruses has been intense, it seems likely that—in this respect at least—humans are more like rats than mice. Certainly, there is no evidence that breast cancer is more common in women who were breast-fed.[52]

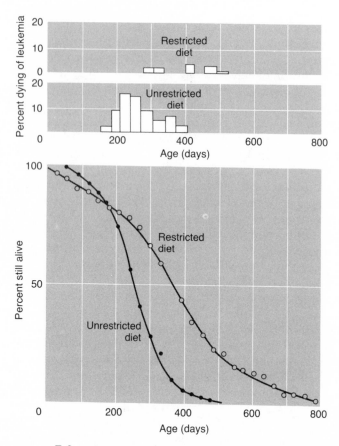

FIGURE 7-9   Murine leukemia and diet. Top: The death rate of a high-leukemia (AK) strain of mice from the spontaneous leukemia produced by murine leukemia virus (MLV) is greatly reduced by restricting their diet. Bottom: As a result the mice live longer and tend eventually to die of other causes. [After J. A. Saxton, M. C. Boon and J. Furth. *Cancer Res.* **4,** 401–409 (1944).]

    The existence of these various viral cancers in animals amply justifies a continuing search for similar viruses that could be causing human cancers; after all, it is not very likely that man should be totally spared such diseases. The most plausible candidate for a human tumor virus is a member of the herpes group called the Epstein-Barr virus (EBV). This is associated with two rare varieties of cancer, Burkitt's lymphoma (which affects children in Africa) and nasopharyngeal carcinoma (which affects old people in Southeast Asia);[53] but the exact nature of the association is rather obscure because infection with the virus is almost universal in these populations, whereas the cancers are extremely rare and can occasionally arise in the absence of virus. The other plausible candidate is a related virus called herpes simplex type II; this virus can be spread venereally[54] and is often found associated with cancer of the uterine cervix;[55] but here too the correlation of virus and cancer is not absolute. As for the major human cancers (such as lung, colon, breast, stomach, and pancreas), there is so far no evidence that viruses are involved.

So much for the natural cancers of man and animals. The difficulties really start when we come to consider what might be called the unnatural cancers. Roughly a quarter of the 200 or 300 known viruses of vertebrates have been shown to be capable of producing cancers in one or more species, usually when inoculated in large quantities into very young animals. To pick just one example, a small DNA virus called polyoma virus is widely distributed among wild and inbred strains of mice. Normally it does not produce any disease even though it can be present in fairly large quantities. However, when it is inoculated into young hamsters or newborn mice it produces tumors in many tissues. Obviously such forms of tumorigenesis are, in the literal sense of the word, artifacts. They have, however, been made the subject of most intense research because it is thought (perhaps correctly) that even if they bear no relationship to the usual process of carcinogenesis they may at least provide an insight into the factors determining the behavior of normal and cancerous cells. For example, polyoma virus is so small that it contains totally only three or four genes, and not even all of these are essential for carcinogenesis; it may be possible therefore to determine the exact function of the one or two virus products needed to transform a cell into a cancer cell, and thereby learn something about carcinogenesis. Such studies on the molecular biology of *in vitro* "transformation," as it is called, will be discussed in the next chapter. It is important, however, not to fall here into the common trap of thinking that cancer must be a virus disease just because these artifactual forms of carcinogenesis are so amenable to analysis.

To complete this section, we must consider how viruses originated in the first place because there is a distinct possibility that some kinds of tumor viruses are themselves artifacts. The essential character of all viruses is that their genetic material, whether RNA or DNA, is translated and replicated by the machinery of the cell they are parasitizing. The larger viruses are thought to have evolved from bacteria that attempted to grow inside cells, be-

came confined to that habitat, and then gradually shed the more
cumbersome parts of their biochemical armory so that they became totally dependent on their host; in contrast, the smaller
viruses, whose nucleic acid is usually closely related to their
host's, are thought to have originated from within the host cell as
clusters of genes that have gained the ability to move from one
cell to another and so have acquired an independent identity. The
evolution of viruses from bacteria does not put too great a strain
on the imagination. But the small viruses are more of a problem
because, as a minimal requirement, they have to contain genes
responsible for making the proteins of the virus coat that protects
the nucleic acid as it moves on to the next cell, plus whatever
genes are required to divert the synthetic machinery of host cells
into making the virus's nucleic acid and proteins. The difficulty is
that these two groups of genes have to come together all at the
same moment, and it is hard to see how that came to pass. The
problem became more acute when it was discovered that certain
small RNA tumor viruses have their RNA transcribed into corresponding chains of DNA, which are then integrated into the DNA
of the host cell.[56] The enzyme responsible for this transcription of
RNA into DNA (*reverse transcriptase* as it is called) is not
commonly present in cells, and so the gene for that enzyme is just
one more item the virus must acquire at the moment of its creation. The necessary concurrence of events now seems so unlikely
that the following ingenious alternative has been proposed (see
also Figure 7-10): the normal development of the different tissues

FIGURE 7-10   The protovirus hypothesis. According to this hypothesis, the
formation of RNA tumor viruses resulted from the accidental juxtaposition of
transcripts of genes for initiation of cell multiplication, genes for certain proteins
involved in the packaging of transcripts, and the gene for reverse transcriptase.
The hypothesis requires that cells already possess the capability for moving their
genes around in this manner. The imagined sequence of events required for
such gene rearrangements is shown in the diagram.

(a) The way in which a set of genes from one region of a cell's DNA (region I)
could be moved to another part of the DNA (region II). First, an RNA transcript of
those genes is made (just like any other messenger). This transcript is then
copied back into DNA (by the enzyme, reverse transcriptase). The resulting DNA
molecule can then be integrated into some distant region of the cell's DNA. In
this way, the genes in that molecule acquire a new context in which to be
expressed.

(b) The creation and spread of new gene combinations (represented here by
the letters) from one cell to another. If the initial RNA transcript were packaged in
a protein shell (i.e., were made into a typical RNA virus particle) it could survive
in the extracellular environment and therefore could be passed from one cell to
another before being copied back into DNA and reintegrated.

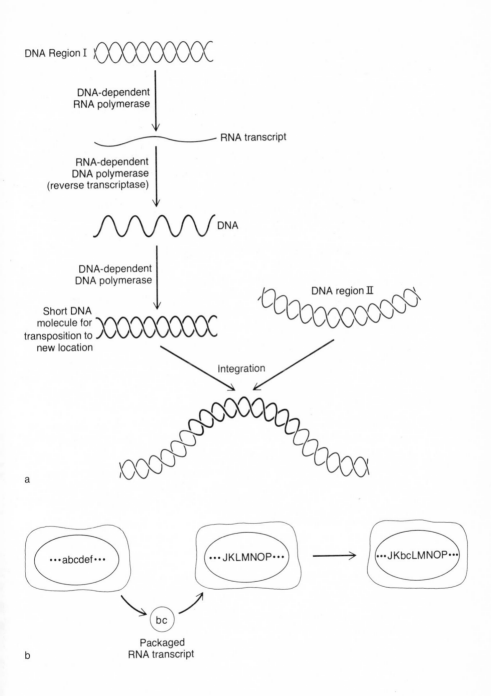

DNA Region I

DNA-dependent
RNA polymerase

RNA transcript

RNA-dependent
DNA polymerase
(reverse transcriptase)

DNA

DNA-dependent
DNA polymerase

DNA region II

Short DNA
molecule for
transposition to
new location

Integration

a

···abcdef···

···JKLMNOP···

···JKbcLMNOP···

bc

Packaged
RNA transcript

b

of multicellular organisms may conceivably require some rearrangement of the genetic message in the different classes of cells and this might be accomplished by mobile sets of genes that travel not only between various regions of a cell's chromosomes but occasionally even from one cell to another; the movement could depend on transcription of genes into RNA and back again, combined with special methods for packaging the message for transport between cells and for integrating that message when it reaches its destination. Such a system could easily evolve because it could develop gradually.

The theory, which is called the *protovirus hypothesis*,[57] is therefore that the RNA tumor viruses are minor aberrations of a device used normally in development. In fact, the argument has been taken one step further with the suggestion that certain of these tumor viruses are actually laboratory artifacts. For example, one of the earliest tumors to be studied was a spontaneous tumor of chickens, the Rous sarcoma; at first it could be transmitted only between closely related chickens (i.e., it could not cross histocompatibility barriers); later, however, the tumor could be transferred with some difficulty by cell-free extracts, and from then on transfer became possible even between species. So it does look rather as if the cancer cell came first and subsequently, because of the intense selection pressure imposed by the histocompatibility barrier, the particular set of genes responsible for the cancer became transferred to a virus that was not subject to any such barrier and could move freely from one animal to another.

The possibility that certain tumor viruses are simply laboratory artifacts makes them in some respects more interesting rather than less, because it means that they may be offering us a way of isolating and studying the genes responsible for the cancerous state. That seems to be the real justification for putting so much effort into investigating the tumor viruses, not the vague hope that human cancer will turn out to be a virus disease.

EXPERIMENTAL
CANCER RESEARCH (2):
THE CANCER CELL

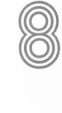

The properties of cancer cells and the methods for creating them from normal cells, cultivated in vitro, *have been investigated most intensively, especially during the last 10 years. The hope is that by studying such "transformation"* in vitro *it may be possible to construct a picture of malignant behavior in terms of molecular biology and then somehow apply this knowledge to the control of human cancer. Far from being difficult to investigate, cells seem to show too many changes during transformation, and it is still not known which if any of the changes are essential to the usual process of carcinogenesis in human beings.*

The preceding chapter was concerned with some of the ways in which cancer may be produced in animals. Once a large array of such experimental cancers were available for study, the next step was obviously to compare the properties of cancer cells and their normal counterparts in the hope of learning what it is that makes them malignant and therefore how they might be brought back under control.

The Cancer Cell *in Vivo*

As pointed out in Chapter 3, the actions of all our cells, particularly their multiplication, are under very strict control. The advent of molecular genetics has inspired a certain confidence that the understanding of cell control is a soluble problem, within the reach of modern technology. We have learned from study of the genes in bacteria how cells, which have inherited the same genetic material, can assume different properties by switching on specific combinations of genes and switching off others. In the absence of strong evidence to the contrary, it seems reasonable to suppose that the mechanisms used for the differentiation of the various classes of vertebrate cells operate in much the same way. For example, the frog egg can undergo normal development as far as the tadpole stage after its own nucleus has been killed by irradiation and replaced by the nucleus of a fully differentiated cell from an adult frog (Figure 8-1);[1] taken at face value, this result implies that differentiated cells still retain all the genes needed to make a tadpole (i.e., that differentiation is accomplished by gene control, not gene loss). If cell behavior is fundamentally determined by gene control, it follows that the abnormal behavior of the cancer cell probably results from some change in the choice of genes that are active within it—either the loss (or repression) of certain genes that exercise a controlling effect, or the activation of genes that normally function only in another class of cell or only at some earlier stage of development. These changes then give the cell a set of properties that are never found together in a normal cell. So, when we try to identify the essential characteristics of a cancer cell, we are probably looking for particular identifiable genes that will prove to be switched on (or off) in cancer cells but not in their normal counterparts.

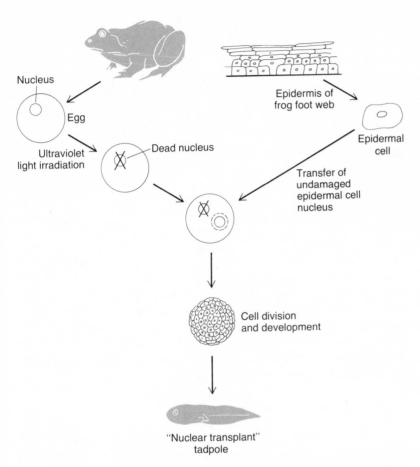

Nucleus

Egg

Epidermis of
frog foot web

Ultraviolet
light irradiation

Dead nucleus

Epidermal
cell

Transfer of
undamaged
epidermal cell
nucleus

Cell division
and development

"Nuclear transplant"
tadpole

FIGURE 8-1   The nuclei of differentiated cells (such as the skin or gut cells of
the frog *Xenopus*) apparently retain the full set of genes necessary for
development of all the tissues of the body. For example, if the development of
the fertilized egg of a frog has been blocked by irradiating its nucleus with
ultraviolet light, the egg can be made to develop (at least to the tadpole stage) by
injecting into it the intact nucleus from a differentiated cell. [After J. B. Gurdon et
al., *J. Embryol. Exp. Morph.* **34,** 93–112 (1975).]

The rate of multiplication of the cells in the body is normally
closely controlled, and precisely matches their rate of loss. In skin
(the example discussed in Chapter 3) the deepest cells divide just
fast enough to replace the cells that are being shed all the time
from the surface, so that the total population of cells remains

constant. The salient feature of the cancer cell is that it is not subject to such precise control and is thus able to create an ever-expanding family of descendants. It is a common mistake to assume that cancer cells multiply faster than the normal cells from which they were derived—for example, that skin cancer cells divide faster than the basal cells in normal skin, and that leukemia cells divide faster than the normal progenitor cells in bone marrow or lymph glands. The fact is that the cells of most cancers divide at about the normal rate, and some even less frequently than their normal counterparts, but they are able to increase in number because a greater proportion of the cells' progeny remain in the dividing pool than is normally allowed.[2]

Normally, the system that controls cell division seems to be some form of spatial restraint. For example, there is a limited layer or zone in the epithelium of the skin[3] and intestine[4] in which cell division is permitted, and once cells are forced outside this compartment they lose the ability to divide, and proceed to embark on their terminal program of differentiation which ends with their dying or being discarded; skin cells form into flakes of keratin and are shed; similarly, the white cells formed by the marrow circulate in the blood for a while and then migrate through the gut wall to be digested.[5] In contrast the cancer cell is less bound by such restraints. Although it usually retains the ability to undergo the kind of terminal differentiation shown by its normal counterpart (e.g., the cells of a skin cancer can still form keratin flakes), it has somehow become able to expand endlessly the size of the compartment in which division is permitted. In other words, its foremost defect may well have something to do with whatever signaling system delineates that compartment.

We see disturbance of the signaling systems clearly demonstrated in the different varieties of breast cancer. The epithelium of the normal female breast is made up of tree-like sets of branching ducts that end in small hollow cell-lined cavities (*alveoli*). Like the trees in a forest, the different branching systems are arrayed in a fairly orderly way and keep their distance from each other. Between neighboring ducts a supporting framework of fibrous tissue and blood vessels (the *stroma*) makes up the main mass of the breast. The whole ordered structure depends on the communication between epithelium and stroma; each dictates the behavior of the other (see p. 31). Judging from the microscopic anatomy of different breast cancers, this communication can be upset in many different ways. Some cancers are composed mainly of proliferating epithelium, as if the cells have partly escaped from the control of the stroma; in others, the tumor may be composed almost entirely of stroma, suggesting that the cancerous epithelium is sending out some abnormal signal which provokes the stroma into excessive growth. In some the cancerous epithelium seems to be trying to form ducts, and in others, alveoli; in still others, the epithelium seems to have lost all form and is made up of very primitive, undifferentiated cells. Some breast cancers retain the normal sensitivity to sex hormones; some do not.

This variation suggests the existence of an intricate system of intercommunication of epithelial cells, with each other and with the underlying stroma, that can be partially interrupted in many different ways. Some simple means of cell communication, for which the mechanism is roughly understood, have been mentioned earlier. But for the most part, we have no idea of the system of signals controlling a structure such as the breast. An obvious exercise is to look for changes in surface proteins that could affect the interactions between cells in direct contact with each other, or to look for changes in the intracellular proteins that act as receptors for general signals like hormones. For example, the surfaces of normal epithelial cells are so arranged that they form a system of intercommunicating channels (called *gap junctions*) whenever they come into contact with each other; cancer cells, however, usually do not form gap junctions either among themselves or, at the edge of a cancer, with their normal neighbors (Figure 8-2).[6] That is one of the few surface changes, observed in cancer cells *in vivo*, that seems likely to have some bearing on their behavior.

So much for the unrestrained multiplication of the cancer cell at the primary site. The next property we must consider is that of invasiveness. However much a group of abnormal cells may grow in number, the tumor they form will be considered benign as long as it is confined to its proper territory and can therefore be easily excised. The first step in malignancy occurs when the cells break out of their normal confines and start to invade the surrounding tissues. The ability to spread is usually accompanied by the ability to enter the circulation of blood or lymph and undergo metastasis to distant sites. At this point the tumor is classified as malignant (i.e., is called a cancer) because its cells can pass beyond the reach of local surgery. Because invasion and metastasis are such dangerous events in the growth of a cancer, great efforts

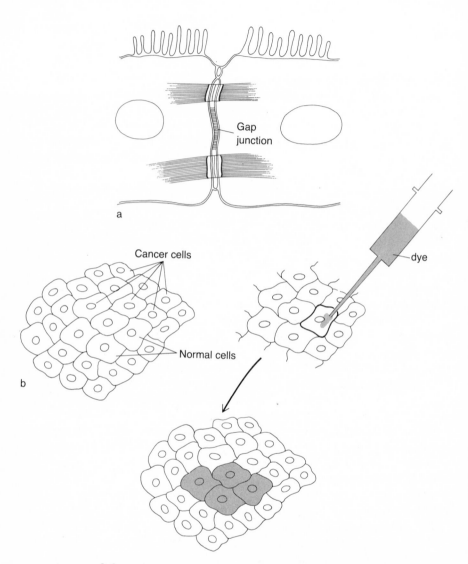

FIGURE 8-2   The absence of close connections between cancer cells. (a) The opposed surfaces of normal epithelial cells make contact with each other at special regions of their surface called *gap junctions* through which small molecules can freely move from one cell to the next; cancer cells do not make such connections either with themselves or with normal cells. (b) As a result, when dye is injected into a normal cell it will spread to any normal neighboring cells but not to any adjoining cancer cells.

have been made to find out what cell properties these processes depend on.

Early in the study of cancer cells cultivated *in vitro,* it was observed that excised pieces of cancers would dissolve clotted blood plasma faster than pieces of normal tissue. Since then many cancer lines have been shown to produce extracellular enzymes that digest proteins (Figure 8-3).[7] Similar enzymes are also produced by certain special cells on the outside of the developing embryo (the *trophoblast* cells) that invade the lining of the uterus to bring about implantation of the fertilized egg, and by certain cells in the adult animal (e.g., the macrophages) whose function is

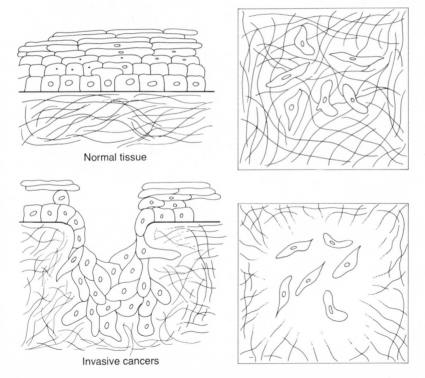

Normal tissue

Invasive cancers

FIGURE 8-3   One factor that may contribute to the invasiveness of cancer cells is their ability to produce extracellular enzymes (e.g., plasminogen activator) that will digest proteins. For example, when cells are cultured *in vitro* (sketches at right) and made to spread out on glass that has been coated with the protein fibrin, normal cells will leave the fibers of fibrin intact, whereas many lines of cancer cells will dissolve the fibers.

to digest dead cells, bacteria, and other foreign bodies. It is conceivable therefore that the character of invasiveness may often result from the activation of genes that normally function only early in the development of the embryo, or only in certain terminally differentiated cells like macrophages that are incapable of prolonged cell division.

Another important property of cancers, essential if they are to grow to any large size, is that they should attract an adequate blood supply. It may be significant that, when transplanted to a normally nonvascular site like the cornea, many cancers will quickly become invaded by blood vessels (Figure 8-4), whereas normal tissues are not. This suggests that cancer cells may be producing diffusible, long-range signals that provoke the growth and migration of normal blood vessels towards them.[8]

Perhaps the most important property of cancers is their ability to undergo metastasis. Normal cells will not multiply at distant, alien sites if injected intravenously or subcutaneously; (this is just as well, because even such a simple procedure as giving a hypodermic injection apparently often introduces a clump of skin cells with whatever is being injected).[9] The reason is not that the cells die, but rather that they lie dormant simply because they are not receiving any signals asking for their division. For example, if the cells from a small piece of a mouse thyroid gland are inoculated intravenously back into the mouse, they settle in the lung

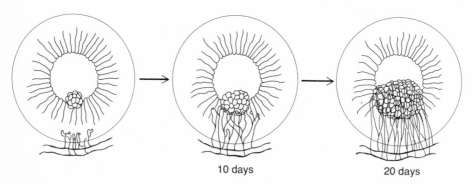

10 days   20 days

FIGURE 8-4   The ability of cancer cells to grow and form large tumors depends partly on their ability to collect an adequate blood supply. When transplanted to relatively nonvascular sites (such as the cornea), most cancers will stimulate an invasion by surrounding blood vessels, whereas blocks of normal tissue will not. [After Folkman, "The Vascularization of Tumors," Copyright 1976 by Scientific American, Inc. All rights reserved.]

but do not multiply (Figure 8-5); however, at any time later in the life of the mouse, these dormant cells can be made to multiply and form deposits in the lungs by feeding the mouse methylthiouracil—a substance known to provoke the pituitary gland into producing an excess of the thyroid-stimulating hor-

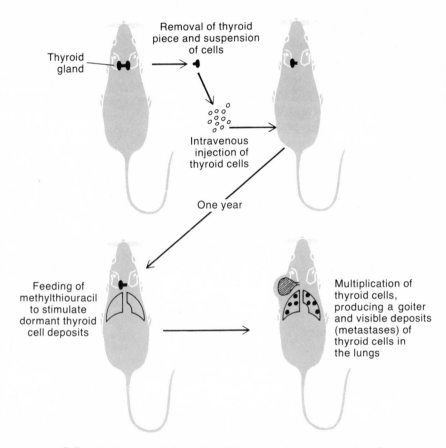

FIGURE 8-5   The fate of cells inoculated intravenously can be most easily determined when they have been derived from an endocrine gland, because it is then possible to test for their continued presence. For example, when normal thyroid cells are inoculated intravenously they are deposited in the lung where they then remain dormant unless stimulated to multiply by the feeding of a substance (such as methylthiouracil) that stimulates the thyroid (note the goiter that results as well). Thus apparently the spread of normal cells throughout the body may be partly prevented simply by the absence of signals that could stimulate the cells to multiply in alien sites.

mone.[10] This experiment suggests that one barrier to metastasis may be the inability of normal cells to grow when removed from the source of any signals prompting their multiplication. In addition, there may also be territorial restraints. For example, in mice, cells capable of colonizing the bone marrow circulate in the bloodstream; yet, as experiments with appropriately marked cells show, these circulating, potentially colonizing cells cannot get a foothold in the marrow because it is already fully occupied, and so the only thing left to them is to undergo terminal differentiation and death.[11] However, if a mouse has been X-irradiated, so that its marrow cells have been destroyed, the marrow can be recolonized by a blood transfusion from an unirradiated mouse.

To create a cell that can undergo metastasis, specificity must be relaxed somewhat. Any cell that normally divides only when it receives the appropriate signal from another class of cell (e.g., an epithelial cell in skin that receives signals from the underlying dermis) must either learn to grow independently or at least acquire a more catholic taste. Some normal cells are more versatile than others. In the rabbit, for example, normal mammary epithelium will form skin if grafted onto the skin surface (i.e., it can respond to signals from the rabbit dermis), but this procedure will not work in the rat.[12]

One of the commonest cancers of human skin is the basal cell carcinoma. Although this is one of the most locally invasive of all cancers, it almost never produces metastases, perhaps because its particular set of defects may make it totally dependent on being accompanied by cells of the dermis. In general, each kind of human cancer tends to spread more to some sites than to others. Cancer of the lung commonly spreads to the brain, for example, and cancer of the breast and prostate tend to spread to bone.[13] Obviously we are going to have to learn much more about the normal interactions between cells of different types, before we can hope to understand much about metastasis.

We can summarize this section in the following way. In order to form a spreading, malignant tumor, the cancer cell must have acquired not one but several unusual properties that distinguish it from its normal counterpart. We might suppose therefore that several steps have to take place during the genesis of a cancer, and this reasoning is certainly supported by epidemiological evidence (see p. 36). One way of dissecting the process further has been to study the properties of cancer cells in culture.

The Cancer Cell *in Vitro*. Transformation

The incentive behind most early attempts to culture mammalian tissues *in vitro* was the wish to compare the properties of normal cells and cancer cells. As a result, a huge literature has accumulated in which the specific study of cancer cells has become inextricably mixed with the general problems of tissue culture.

Not every class of mammalian cell can be easily propagated *in vitro*. The reason is probably that most cells in the body belong to mixed groups consisting of several mutually interdependent cell classes, and so one should not expect one such class to flourish on its own. In fact, it has seldom been possible to set up growing cultures from naturally arising cancers and from their normal noncancerous equivalents for purposes of comparing their properties. Far more successful has been the study of the growth of normal cells *in vitro* and of the ways of converting them into cancer cells that will form tumors when transplanted back into animals.

When small pieces of tissue are placed in a culture vessel, such as a Petri dish, and covered with a nutrient medium containing serum, the cells that grow best are a highly selected population thought to be derived from the blood vessels in the tissue, but because of their appearance they have come to be known as *fibroblasts*.[14] These cells will multiply and spread out over the floor of the culture vessel much faster than any other class of cell, hence they quickly take over; for this reason, until fairly recently most of the cultured cells (cell lines) that people worked with were made up of fibroblasts. As the growing fibroblasts spread out and cover the entire floor of the culture vessel, they eventually exhaust their supply of nutrients and stop multiplying. At that point the usual laboratory practice is to detach the cells by treating them with the proteolytic enzyme trypsin, and seed a few of the detached cells into fresh containers where they can settle down and start multiplying again.

The first unexpected finding was that, for many cell lines, this process of serial transfer cannot be repeated indefinitely.[15] For example, most lines of human fibroblasts die out after the cells have divided about 50 times. In fact, much the same effect is seen when whole tissues, such as skin or mammary gland, are transplanted serially from one animal to another; for example, some mouse tissues can be kept multiplying for about three times the normal mouse's lifespan before they die out.[16] However, it is conceivable that cell division really has no set limit, and that cultures of fibroblasts (and other classes of cell) would not die out if they had been properly looked after and given all the right growth factors.[17]

This might seem like an academic argument, were it not for the phenomenon of spontaneous transformation.[18] When the fibroblasts of certain species are continually cultivated, variants can arise that have a somewhat altered style of growth and prove to be exempt from aging (meaning that they can be cultivated indefinitely). Instead of being spread flat on the floor of the culture vessel, they are more rounded and will grow to form colonies in which the cells are heaped one upon another. This change, which is called *transformation*, imparts to the transformed colony a considerable survival advantage in the final stages of growth, and so the transformed cells eventually come to dominate the culture. These are the cells that make up what are called *permanent*, or *established*, cell lines. Now, when cultured mouse fibroblasts are injected back into the mouse strain from which they were derived, they will often form tumors if they have undergone transformation, but usually not otherwise. This argues rather strongly that some of the steps in carcinogenesis may affect the processes that normally lead to aging. (Actually the correlation of transformation, immortality, and tumorigenicity is less than perfect, because some permanent established cell lines have not undergone a morphological transformation, and of these lines some are tumorigenic in animals and some are not.)[19]

The same kind of transformation can be produced by exposing cultured cells to various chemicals and viruses that are known to cause cancer in animals, and such transformed cells tend to be tumorigenic. It is thought by many that this transformation is in fact the process of carcinogenesis being enacted under controllable conditions, and that it should be possible with modern technology to find out exactly what the various carcinogens are doing.

However it is necessary to sound a word of caution about these experimental results before we discuss transformation further. The appearance of spontaneously transformed variants is very common when mouse cells are being cultivated, rather rare for hamster and rat cells, and virtually unknown for human and chicken cells. This difference between the cells of different species turns out to be crucial to the study of carcinogenesis *in vitro*. Cells

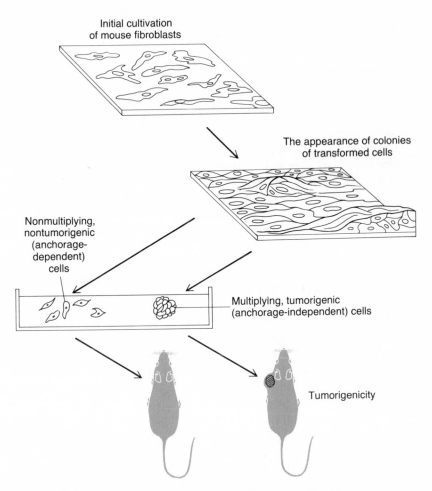

Initial cultivation
of mouse fibroblasts

The appearance of colonies
of transformed cells

Nonmultiplying,
nontumorigenic
(anchorage-
dependent)
cells

Multiplying, tumorigenic
(anchorage-independent) cells

Tumorigenicity

FIGURE 8-6   Spontaneous Transformation. When mouse fibroblasts are cultivated *in vitro*, cell variants frequently arise that grow as heaped-up colonies. These "transformed" cells are capable of multiplying when suspended in agar (i.e., they have acquired what is called *anchorage independence*) and are often able to form progressively growing tumors when inoculated back into mice.

that undergo spontaneous transformation can be transformed into tumorigenic cells *in vitro* fairly efficiently by tumor viruses, irradiation, and chemical carcinogens. Cells such as human and chicken cells, which hardly ever undergo spontaneous transformation *in vitro*, can be transformed by viruses but not easily by irradiation or by chemical carcinogens.[20]

It is tempting to think that these differences in susceptibility to physical and chemical transformation may conceivably be related to lifespan. Mice and men are exposed to much the same levels of radiation and mutagenic chemicals, but human cells have to withstand becoming transformed for 30 times as long as mouse cells. How they do this is not known. There seems to be no great difference in the mutability of human and mouse cells by a given dose of mutagen,[21] and so the stronger resistance of human cells to transformation may depend on the way their controls are organized. For example, human cells may be hedged in with more controls than mouse cells, so that more genes must be mutated or derepressed to transform them than to transform mouse cells. Certainly, until the difference between the transformability of long- and short-lived species is understood, we should be cautious in applying to man the results of experiments with rodent cells.

Transformation by Viruses

In recent years, a long list of agents have been shown to transform cells *in vitro* and make them capable of forming tumors when inoculated back into animals. Many of the chemicals known to be carcinogenic will do this,[22] as will ultraviolet light[23] and X-irradiation.[24] But by far the most popular agents for producing *in vitro* transformation are the tumor viruses. The reasoning behind their popularity seems to have been as follows. The final object of studying cancer cells and carcinogenesis *in vitro* is to determine the exact ways in which the cancer cell is altered. In principle, this could be achieved by picking a representative set of cancers produced by a suitably wide range of carcinogens, and then comparing these cells with normal cells in every possible, measurable parameter; but in practice this indiscriminate approach has not been very rewarding. The number of things that could be measured is just too large; after all, each cell contains the products of many thousands of genes. So what is needed is some way of improving the odds. One way has been to examine what is most likely to have changed, namely the cell surface. Another has been to study transformation by agents that, because of their nature, can be singled out and observed during their interaction with a cell, namely the tumor viruses.

About a quarter of all known viruses of vertebrates have been shown to be capable of producing tumors in animals.[25] But by far the greatest amount of work has been done with certain very small viruses,[26] in particular two DNA-containing viruses, polyoma and SV40, and a group of RNA-containing viruses, of which Rous sarcoma virus is the prototype. These viruses are so small that they contain only three or four genes, and therefore it is feasible to consider subjecting them to a complete chemical analysis—i.e., determining the entire sequence of bases in their nucleic acid, and the exact structure and function of each of their gene products. With that information in hand, we might hope to determine exactly what the virus does when it transforms a cell into a cancer cell. This chemical marathon will be completed in the next year or two, but it has already become clear that the small tumor viruses exhibit many interesting features in their interaction with cells during transformation. These are best exemplified by polyoma virus and Rous sarcoma virus.

Polyoma virus is widespread in mice, both in laboratory strains and in the wild. It was discovered accidentally about 25 years ago when attempts to transfer murine leukemia to infant mice by inoculating cell-free filtrates of leukemic tissue unexpectedly produced tumors of the salivary glands. Subsequently the virus was purified free of leukemia virus and shown to be capable of producing a wide range of tumors in many species of rodents (hence the name *polyoma,* meaning many tumors), although there is no indication that it ever produces tumors under natural conditions, in which the virus arrives in a low dose and is not inoculated. When susceptible cells are exposed to polyoma virus, two responses are possible. The virus may multiply in the cell nucleus, until eventually the cell dies and liberates the new virus particles formed within it; this has been called the productive or lytic response and is the way the virus grows and survives in nature; the cell is not transformed but dies. Less commonly, the virus may for some reason not be extensively replicated, but its DNA becomes incorporated (integrated) into the cell's DNA, where it remains forever afterwards, like any set of cellular genes, being faithfully copied and transferred to all the cell's descendants; this is the response that leads to transformation. By studying various mutants of the virus, defective in different genes, it has been possible to show that at least two out of the three or four genes in the virus are not essential for transformation. The remaining gene (or genes) is essential for the act of transformation and also probably for maintaining the transformed state. The function of the gene is apparently to switch on host DNA synthesis and, in productive infections, also switch on the synthesis of viral DNA.

There are several ways in which the presence of the virus might bring about the changes in cell behavior that accompany transformation (Figure 8-7). One possibility is that the changes are the direct consequence of integrating the viral DNA into the cell's DNA.[27] Classical studies of the genetics of plants and bacteria have shown that the general arrangement of a cell's DNA can determine which genes are active: for example, a gene that is normally repressed can be dragged into action by the insertion of an active gene next to it (Figure 8-7a), or conversely be repressed by the insertion of such a gene (Figure 8-7b); and obviously, an active gene will be made non-functional if a stretch of alien DNA is inserted in its midst (Figure 8-7c); we might imagine therefore that the rare occasions on which polyoma virus produces trans-

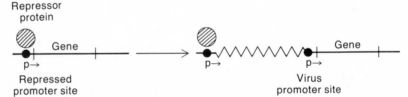

(a) Integration of virus DNA (⌇⌇) provides a new, unrepressed promoter site (p→) for messenger RNA synthesis so that transcription of a neighboring, normally repressed cellular gene can take place.
Result: The cell gains another protein.

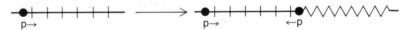

(b) Integration of virus DNA introduces a promoter site (←p) that causes backwards transcription of neighboring cellular genes, and the enzymes carrying out this transcription collide with and block the enzymes doing the normal forward transcription of these genes.
Result: The cell loses one or more of its proteins.

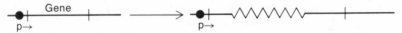

(c) Integration of virus DNA into the middle of a cellular gene breaks up the message.
Result: The cell loses one of its proteins.

FIGURE 8-7   Some of the possible ways in which viruses, such as polyoma, may change cells when they become integrated into the cells' DNA.

formation are those where the virus DNA integrates near, or actually within, some gene whose function is crucial for controlling cell behavior. If so, the virus may indicate for us which genes are involved in carcinogenesis. Unfortunately, it turns out, at least when SV40 (a virus closely related to polyoma) is integrated, that different lines of transformed cells prove to contain virus DNA integrated into different regions of the cell DNA, suggesting that no single cellular gene will be found to be directly affected in all transformed cells.[28] This essentially negative result is something of a setback for those who had hoped that identifying the integration site used by these viruses would lead to a quick solution to the cancer problem.

Another completely different possibility (not shown in Figure 8-7) is that transformation involves a protein coded by one of the virus genes. This protein is called the Tumor antigen, or T antigen, and can be detected in all cells containing polyoma virus. There is good evidence that it has an essential function both in the initiation and in the maintenance of the transformed state;[29] thus virus that has undergone a mutation making the T antigen unstable at high temperature is unable to transform cells at that temperature. Some idea of the possible function of the T antigen comes from studying the timing of events after transformation. Transformed mouse (or hamster) lines will generally not form tumors immediately following transformation; after a few weeks of cultivation *in vitro*, a million cells may have to be implanted into a mouse in order for a tumor to arise, but within a month or two the critical dose may have fallen to a thousand.[30] Other changes, such as abnormalities in the number or appearance of the chromosomes, develop in parallel. Where polyoma is the transforming agent, it may therefore turn out to be misleading to think of transformation as the end of the road leading to tumorigenesis. Instead the integrated virus and its T antigen may act simply by stimulating cell division and it may be this that promotes the eventual appearance of a tumorigenic cell line.

The other virus we should consider is Rous sarcoma virus (RSV). It is one member of a large family of RNA-containing viruses that can produce tumors in various species. The viruses fall into two groups, according to the type of tumor they produce. The leukemia viruses, such as feline leukemia virus (FeLV), cause leukemias in natural animal populations, but are generally unable to transform cells in culture. The sarcoma viruses, such as RSV, will readily transform almost any species of cell but although they produce sarcomas in experimental animals they are found rarely, if at all, outside the laboratory. Indeed, as pointed out on p. 118, they probably originated in the laboratory when certain cellular genes that are capable of making cells tumorigenic became incorporated into a virus. Like polyoma, these viruses contain only a few genes and so there is a limit to how complicated a life they can lead, but in almost every other respect they are completely different from polyoma. Their nucleic acid is RNA, not DNA, and so it can be translated directly in the cell to make viral proteins but it cannot be integrated into the cell's DNA until it has been transcribed into DNA.

Transformation and the production of progeny virus by RSV (or other RNA tumor viruses) are not mutually exclusive, as they are in polyoma. Indeed, RSV-transformed cells continually liberate virus particles and this is crucial to their tumorigenicity because it allows them to recruit more and more cells into the tumor.[31] As in polyoma virus, at least one of the genes in RSV is essential for the initiation and maintenance of transformation. But the remarkable feature of the essential gene in RSV is that it (or a very closely related gene) is also found in the normal non-transformed cells of many species.[32] This gene is called sarc (short for sarcoma) and its association with both cells and viruses might be explained in the following way. There may be many genes actively concerned with cell proliferation that are used during development of the embryo but are not expressed during adult life. If one of these genes happens by accident to be transcribed into RNA at a time when the cell is also making a virus like RSV, then the RNA transcript of the gene could become joined to the viral RNA and carried with it forever afterwards. Later, when a cell is infected with this composite virus and translates the RNA back into DNA, the cell will therefore find itself with an unrepressed copy of a gene whose function is to bring on cell proliferation, and so it starts to multiply. Obviously this idea is closely related to the protovirus hypothesis for the origin of RSV that was mentioned at the end of the preceding chapter.

Polyoma virus and RSV are the simplest tumor viruses. Less is known about the more complicated viruses, although it is clear that some of them integrate into the cell's DNA during transformation and others do not. Needless to say, the molecular biology of all these viruses is proving such an engrossing subject that it is easy to forget that the object of the exercise is to learn something about the origin and characteristics of the transformed cell, and this is the topic of the following section.

The Transformed Cell

The obvious distinguishing feature of transformed cells, whether arising spontaneously or produced by chemicals or viruses, is that they grow into heaped up colonies of rather rounded cells piled one upon another in a disordered array. Normal cells are usually angular and tidily arranged and tend to stop growing when they touch each other. The transformed cell's lack of order and loss of restraint are what one might expect of a cancer cell, but it is still not clear which of the chemical changes that commonly accompany transformation are causes and which are effects.

The ability to grow at high cell concentration (the loss of *contact inhibition*, or *density-dependent regulation* as it is now called) is partly due to a decreased requirement for a variety of growth factors that are normally present in serum and gradually become depleted from culture media as the cells increase in number.[33] In the past few years, a bewildering array of such factors have been isolated from serum, but it is not clear which of them are important for regulating growth *in vivo*. Certainly it seems likely that most cells in the body are responding at any given moment to a large number of different signals, and so the existence of a plethora of control substances should not surprise us.

What makes a transformed cell less demanding for growth factors is not known. Here we enter a very complex area. A cell can be likened to an elaborate factory that makes many different products, each of which has to be kept in a proper balance with all the others. Because every major policy decision in such a factory affects the action of each production line, an efficient system of communication must be set up between the different departments. We can observe this kind of communication occurring inside cells.[34] For example, when nutrients become in short supply, cells show a particular pattern in the way they shut down their different production lines. This reaction is called the *pleiotypic response* (literally a response characterized by more than one effect) because it bears on many different departments of the cell. It is presumably designed to ensure that all production lines can be started again when the crisis is over. Other similar programmed patterns of behavior have been observed, as for example when cells that are duplicating their DNA meet a chemically altered base in the DNA chain that cannot be copied.

Now, the existence of these complex programs makes it hard to determine which is the fundamental change or defect that underlies the behavior of any particular transformed cell and which are part of the response. To persevere with our industrial metaphor, we can imagine one factory failing because it ceased to respond sensibly to fluctuations in sales, another because it had poor labor relations and a third because it did not maintain its plant properly; despite the difference in their underlying defects, the three could show the same pile-up of uncompleted products halfway along one of the production lines. A simple catalog of the aberrations of the factories (or of the transformed cells) will not necessarily demonstrate the basic defect. In fact, to judge from the example of SV40-transformed cells, it seems probable that each transformed cell is defective in its own particular way.

Apart from an ability to grow at high cell densities, the other obvious property of transformed cells is their altered shape. Normal cells become rounded at the moment of cell division, and in many respects the transformed cell behaves rather as if it were stuck in that state the whole time. For example, various cell surface proteins, that disappear or are covered up during cell division, are present in reduced quantities in almost all transformed cells;[35] similarly, the fluidity of the surface membrane of a transformed cell is increased and is more like that of a cell during the act of division; last, the network of contractile fibers that crisscross the cell and determine its shape and movement are very disorganized, here too like those of a normal cell that is about to divide.[36]

The final and most important property of transformed cells is their ability to form tumors when inoculated back into animals. Although not every transformed cell line shows this property, it is notable that when tumorigenic, transformed lines revert to normal behavior *in vitro* (something that happens very occasionally) they often lose their tumorigenicity. One property of the cells that correlates particularly well with tumorigenesis is their ability to grow in the absence of any solid substratum.[37] Transformed cells will form colonies when suspended in agar (i.e., their growth is *anchorage-independent*); nontransformed cells will not. This *anchorage dependence* of nontransformed cells is plainly important in preventing them from forming tumors, because it has proved possible to produce tumors with one particular, normally nontumorigenic line by inoculating the cells after first sticking them on to glass beads; so the only thing that cell line needs is help in getting started, and it can then form tumors perfectly well (i.e., it has already become somewhat abnormal during prolonged cultivation, even though it is not overtly transformed).[38] Unfortunately, most natural cancers of animals are not readily cultivated by any method, whether offered anchorage or not, so that it is not possible to determine whether loss of anchorage dependence is an important part of their makeup.

We may now return to our starting point in this discussion of the process of transformation and the properties of the transformed cell. The hope is that by studying transformation *in vitro* it may be possible to construct a picture of malignant behavior in molecular terms and then somehow turn this knowledge to use in the control of human cancer. Far from being difficult to discover properties that are peculiar to transformed cells, it has turned out ironically that there are too many changes during transformation, and it is still not known which if any of the changes are important. Indeed, it now seems likely that there is no single entity that one can call "the transformed cell" and no single mystery waiting to be unraveled.

There is one method that should show whether different tumor cells ever share the same defect. It is possible in various ways to make pairs of cells fuse *in vitro* to form hybrids with a double set of chromosomes.[39] Any two tumor cells that had the same set of tumor genes should make a tumorigenic hybrid; whereas cells with different tumor genes might each compensate for the other and therefore make a hybrid that was nontumorigenic (provided, of course, that tumor genes are recessive, and this could be tested by making hybrids with normal cells). Furthermore, as such hybrids tend to shed their excess chromosomes on continued cultivation, it should be possible to pin down exactly which chromosomes carry the genes that make a cell tumorigenic. Unfortunately, the results of such experiments have been confusing. In some situations the ability to form tumors appears to be dominant;[40] in others, it appears to be recessive and, indeed, may remain repressed in a tumor-cell/normal-cell hybrid even when all the normal cell's chromosomes have been lost.[41] So the analysis of the genetics of malignancy by hybridization may turn out to be more complicated than people had hoped.

A few varieties of human cancer, however, have recently been shown, in nearly all cases, to result from some particular genetic defect.[42] In the past few years, ways for distinguishing each of the 23 pairs of human chromosomes have been found, allowing a much more detailed study of the state of the chromosomes in cancer cells. For example, it is now clear that the cells of one form of leukemia (chronic myeloid leukemia) usually exhibit the same chromosomal rearrangement, in which one chromosome-22 is considerably shortened (resulting in the very small *Philadelphia chromosome*, as it is called) because part of it has become translocated to the end of a chromosome-9.[43] Similar regularly recurring rearrangements have been detected in other cancers (e.g., some other forms of leukemia,[44] some cases of breast cancer,[45] Burkitt's lymphoma,[46] and so on); in time more examples will surely be found. It now remains to be determined whether chromosomal rearrangements, perhaps (like insertion sequences, see p. 84) on too small a scale to be detectable by gross microscopy, are a common feature of most cancers.

The Immune Response to Cancer Cells

The function of the immune system is to recognize alien substances entering the body and eliminate them. This is how we are protected against infection by bacteria and viruses, and why we can only accept skin grafts from identical twins. The system operates partly by forming circulating antibodies and partly by producing specifically primed killer cells, but each individual antibody molecule or killer cell is directed against some absolutely specific target (antigen) that the system has decided is not a substance normally present in the body; in other words, the system is set up to distinguish between "self" and "not-self."[47]

The discoverers of the immune system, at the turn of the century, wondered whether one of its functions could be to identify and destroy any incipient cancer cells as fast as they arise;[48] if so, the development of cancer would simply indicate the failure of the normal process of "immune surveillance." The difficulty these early workers had in transplanting tumors from one animal to another, which we now know was due to histocompatibility antigens (see p. 64), lent some support to this concept and led to a lot of very confusing experiments on the immunization of animals against each other's tumors. The present status of such research may be summarized as follows.

The cancer cells produced by tumor viruses do indeed carry novel antigens on their surface that are characteristic for each virus and can be recognized as "not-self" and provoke an immune response.[49] Further, if an animal is incapable of producing this response because of some inherited or imposed defect in its immune system, it will indeed be far more susceptible to almost every kind of tumor virus.[50] Conversely, an animal that has become immunized to a tumor virus without developing a tumor can become resistant; for example, cats that produce only a weak immune response to feline leukemia virus may go on to develop leukemia, whereas those that produce large amounts of antibody do not.[51] It does seem therefore that the immune system functions as a protective device against cancers caused by viruses.

The importance of the immune response against cells transformed by chemical carcinogens is much less clear. Certain chemical carcinogens (e.g., methylcholanthrene, which is one of the active components of coal tar) when given in large doses will produce cancer cells that bear novel antigens on their surface which can induce a specific immune response. However, each tumor apparently bears a unique antigen and evokes a unique, specific immune response; it is possible, for example, to show that a mouse bearing a skin tumor produced by methylcholanthrene is quite resistant to transplants of its own tumor but will accept transplants of another mouse's tumor.[52] In general, however, cancer cells produced experimentally by low doses of chemical carcinogens or arising spontaneously do not seem to evoke a strong immune response.[53] Furthermore, there is no evidence that the immune system can retard the process of chemical carcinogenesis, because animals with defective immune systems are seldom more susceptible to chemical carcinogens.[54]

In recent years it has become possible to test whether immune surveillance is important in the development of human cancers, because we can pick out several groups of people who are known to have an abnormal immune system—either deficient or overreactive—and investigate whether they have a changed incidence of cancer. For example, the recipients of kidney transplants have to be continually treated with drugs that depress the immune response so that they will not reject their transplant.[55] Other people have various inherited defects in their immune system.[56] Then, many of the very old show quite marked immunological unresponsiveness to various test antigens.[57] Finally, besides those with depressed immune systems, there are people whose immune system seems to be overreactive; they are the sufferers from diseases like asthma.[58] The results of surveying these various groups seem absolutely conclusive. Certain very rare cancers affecting cells of the immune system itself are indeed more common in people with immune deficiency, but the common cancers—with a few possible exceptions—are not more common in people with deficiencies in their immune system or less common in overreactive people; (the possible exceptions are cancer of the skin, lip, and cervix, but it is known that cancer of these sites is much more common in the population at large than might be expected from the number of cases that come to the attention of doctors,[59] and so it is hard to calculate how many of these cancers one would expect to find in any closely scrutinized group of people).

This result leads to the conclusion that most of the common human cancers are not subject to immune surveillance:[60] furthermore, since the common human wart[61] and the experimental cancers produced by viruses are made worse by immune suppression whereas the major human cancers are not, we may reasonably deduce that few human cancers are due to viruses. Nevertheless, one can see why the idea of immune surveillance continues to exercise a hypnotic fascination.

Because the crucial abnormality of cancer cells lies in the way they interact with their surroundings, we may expect them to have abnormal surface properties. Indeed, some kinds of cancer cell bear unusual antigens on their surface that are normally found only on proliferating cells in the embryo [62] (this finding lends support to the idea that some of the properties of cancer cells may be due to the expression of those genes that are normally used only during development of the embryo and are dangerously inappropriate in the adult animal). One such surface antigen is the so-called *carcinoembryonic* antigen (CEA), which is found in fetal gut tissue and in the blood of people with advanced cancer of the colon and certain other diseases; another is alpha-fetoprotein, which is found in fetal liver and in the blood of people with liver cancer and certain other tumors. Although those two particular antigens have proved not to be sufficiently specific,[63] it is conceivable that the presence of antigens like these might one day be used as early diagnostic tests for the different kinds of cancer.

The TIME COURSE
of CANCER

9

The process of carcinogenesis appears to be spread throughout much of our lifespan and often seems to proceed through several intermediate, precancerous stages. Different carcinogens probably tend to accelerate different steps in the sequence. If each type of cancer usually has several causes, there may be several ways in which it could be prevented. Understanding the time course of cancer is therefore important not only for the design of screening programs to advance the moment of diagnosis, but also for plans to prevent cancer.

We must now turn from laboratory models of cancer to a more detailed consideration of the process of carcinogenesis in humans. The rapid transformation of cells *in vitro* by agents like Rous sarcoma virus is the kind of reaction readily amenable to investigation; that is one of the reasons why tumor viruses have attracted so much attention. But perhaps the most conspicuous feature of carcinogenesis *in vivo*, in man and experimental animals, is that the process seems normally to extend over a large part of the natural lifespan of the host. This chapter treats various aspects of the time course of carcinogenesis and ends with a brief discussion of the use of screening programs to advance the time of diagnosis.

The Time Course for Development of Human Cancers

For most human cancers, the interval between the first carcinogenic stimulus and the final appearance of the tumor tends to be decades rather than months or years.

This is seen most clearly for those cancers where the exact timing of the initial stimulus is known. For example, after X-irradiation (either therapeutic or diagnostic, or resulting from exposure to the explosion of an atom bomb) the first cancer to appear is leukemia, which reaches its peak incidence about 7 years later (Figure 9-1); by contrast, the commoner kinds of cancer, like breast cancer, do not start to increase in incidence for 10 or 20 years but they probably remain high from then on.[1] A particularly clear-cut but fortunately rare example of a cancer arising long after a limited period of carcinogenesis is the vaginal cancer of girls in their late teens who were exposed to high levels of estrogens *in utero*, when their mothers were treated with stilbestrol to prevent miscarriage.[2] An even longer latent period can be deduced for cancer of the penis: the probability of developing this rare cancer is reduced almost to zero by circumcision, provided that it is carried out in infancy or early childhood; but the cancer that arises in men who are uncircumcised or were not circumcised until they were 10 to 15 years of age does not appear until old age (i.e., after a latent period of 50 years or more).[3] A similar long-delayed response to carcinogenesis in youth is sometimes seen in experimental animals; for example, when four-month-old hamsters are inoculated with SV40 virus (which is

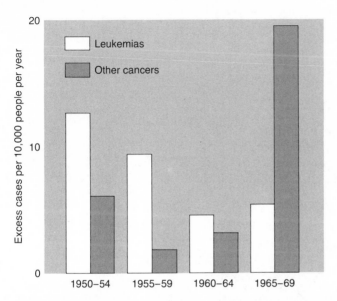

FIGURE 9-1   The time course of appearance of cancer after irradiation. The people who were heavily irradiated in the atom bomb explosions of 1945 (receiving a dose of more than 200 rads) suffered an early increase in incidence of leukemia and, 20 years later, are starting to show an increase in other forms of cancer. [After S. Jablon and H. Kato. *Radiat. Res.* **50,** 649–698, (1972).]

closely related to polyoma), local tumors do not develop for about two years, at which time a hamster is well into old age.[4]

Even when the cause of a cancer cannot be pinned down precisely, it may still be possible to deduce that the process of carcinogenesis extends over a long period of time. For example, the sooner a woman has her first child the lower her chance of having breast cancer in old age;[5] this means that there must be factors operating soon after puberty that will determine the incidence of cancer more than 40 years later. A similar general conclusion comes from the study of migrant populations (see p. 50); for example, the fact that children who migrate to Israel exhibit in old age an overall cancer incidence between the indigenous rate for Israel and the rate characteristic of their country of origin suggests that some of the stimuli for the cancers they have in old age must actually have occurred in their childhood.

In many instances, where human cancers can be attributed to a distinct, identifiable agent, this agent has usually operated continually over a long period of time. As pointed out in Chapter 4, prolonged exposure to industrial carcinogens seldom produces cancer in less than 10 years. Similarly, you have to smoke cigarettes for many years before the risk of lung cancer becomes very high.

Judging from a few well studied examples, it seems that each kind of carcinogen acts by accelerating some of the steps in the production of a cancer and not others. For instance, as Figure 9-2 shows, when people stop smoking, the subsequent annual incidence of lung cancer does not drop but, instead, remains frozen at the approximate level it had reached when they stopped; this suggests that the final step in the sequence occurs at the same

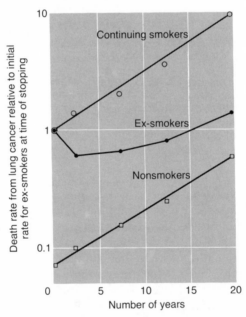

FIGURE 9-2   The relative risk of lung cancer among people who have stopped smoking cigarettes, those who continue to smoke, and those who have never smoked. The annual death rate from lung cancer among a group of British doctors who had stopped smoking was observed for several years. On the basis of British national data for smokers and nonsmokers, the doctors' death rate could then be compared to the expected death rates for two hypothetical groups—one of continuing smokers, the other of nonsmokers—with the same age distribution. The death rates for all three groups are expressed in relation to the rate prevailing for the ex-smokers at the time they stopped. [After R. Doll. *Scot. Med. J.* **15,** 433–447 (1970).]

rate whether you are still smoking or not (i.e., smoking provokes some steps and not others). A similar conclusion has been reached from observing the interaction of different carcinogens. For example, in people who are exposed to asbestos and also happen to smoke, the increase in lung cancer risk proves to be the product rather than the sum of the increments in risk conferred by each agent on its own;[6] this shows that asbestos and smoking activate different steps in the route to lung cancer. At first sight these arguments may seem rather difficult to grasp, but much the same conclusion has come from study of experimental carcinogenesis; recall that in Chapter 6 several examples were given in which one agent (the initiator) was found to provoke early steps in the sequence and a second agent (the promoter) acted on later steps.

Apart from what it tells us about the nature of carcinogenesis, the idea of separate steps driven by separate factors is likely to be very important in the prevention of cancer. If most forms of cancer have several different causes, each tending to act at some particular point in our lives, a policy of prevention could be implemented in a number of ways. To take just one example, most of the lung cancers seen in people who have worked with asbestos could have been prevented if the asbestos industry had refused to employ anyone who smoked (though of course this would not have prevented the other diseases caused by asbestos).

The idea that there are usually several stages in the development of any cancer has another important consequence. Even if we know nothing about the causes of each step in the sequence, it might still be possible to interrupt the progression if there were some way of detecting the intermediate stages. It is of practical importance therefore to discover if any of these stages are associated with visible changes.

Precursor States in Human Cancer

The cancers that are easiest to detect in their early stages are naturally those that occur in the skin. Although they are very common, especially in light-skinned people living in sunny climates, they are not a major cause of mortality because they are mostly very slow-growing and seldom undergo metastasis. Of the human cancers that can be detected at an early stage, the one that causes the greatest mortality is cancer of the uterine cervix, which accounts for roughly 2% of all cancer deaths in Western nations. Because this cancer has been the subject of extensive surveys and screening programs, it is the best example to cite when discussing what is known about precursor states.

At the junction of vagina and uterus (the neck of the uterus, or cervix) the arrangement of the cells in the surface epithelium changes.[7] Externally, as in the rest of the vagina, the cells form a many-layered (*stratified*) epithelium like that of the skin (see p. 26) in which the cells, as they are pushed to the surface, become flattened, lose their nuclei, and are shed like scales. At the immediate entrance to the uterus the arrangement changes to one in which the cells are elongated and form columns lying at right angles to the plane of the surface; this *columnar* epithelium is usually only one or two cells deep, and the cells at the surface are not undergoing the kind of rapid, programmed cell death that is occurring in the neighboring stratified epithelium.

Cancer of the cervix originates in the stratified epithelium, usually very close to its junction with the columnar epithelium of the cervical canal.[8] Why it should be confined to that particular region of the epithelium is unknown, but at least this fact makes it easy to study the changes that precede the appearance of the cancer. Several methods have been used. Cells can be scraped from the epithelium and observed microscopically (this is the familiar "Pap" smear, named after the cytologist Papanicolaou); or quite large samples of the epithelium can be excised and studied microscopically or cultured *in vitro* so that the program of cell renewal can be observed; last, the intact surface can be observed directly.

As a result of mass routine screening, many abnormalities have been described, ranging from minor variations in the developmental pattern of the epithelium, through more severe changes (the so-called carcinoma *in situ*), to invasive metastasizing cancer.[9] Minor changes, such as abnormal thickening of the epithelium or some drift in the boundary between columnar and stratified epithelium, are rather common. The next level of abnormality is called *dysplasia* (literally, "false structuring"); at this stage the cells vary in size and arrangement in a rather haphazard fashion from one area to another, and dividing cells are no longer confined to the deepest layer but are scattered throughout most layers of the epithelium[10] as if they are no longer receiving precise enough positional information to multiply and differentiate in a completely ordered manner. The next level of abnormality is called carcinoma *in situ*; here the signs of differentiation may be minimal, and the only microscopic feature distinguishing the situation from a fully developed cancer is that the dividing line between epithelium and underlying connective tissue is still precisely maintained. Finally, when the abnormal epithelium is seen to be invading the underlying tissues, the condition is classified as a cancer, irrespective of its size or of the detailed appearance of its cells; it is these locally invasive cell populations that are capable of entering lymph and blood vessels and thereby undergoing metastasis to distant sites.

These successive abnormalities, illustrated in Figure 9-3, look very like the successive stages of a sequence; indeed, both dysplasia and carcinoma *in situ* are known to be followed sometimes by the development of a fully invasive cancer. Judging from surveys of women of all ages, the timing is as follows:[11] dysplasia tends to arise at about the age of 30 and persist for 10 to 20 years; carcinoma *in situ* arises rather later and persists for five to 10 years; finally, invasive cancer does not reach maximum incidence until after the age of 60, although it has usually been present and detectable by screening for one to four years before it starts to produce symptoms.

It has proved surprisingly difficult to find out exactly how often these different precursor states actually progress to cancer, and it is not easy to calculate how many lives would be saved by a screening program. The trouble is that it is clear, both from studying the age distribution of the various abnormal states and from observing what happens to women who are not treated,[12] that dysplasia and carcinoma *in situ* are not at all uncommon and usually undergo spontaneous regression; (incidentally, there have been occasional reports of other varieties of cancer undergoing complete regression,[13] but this is a very rare phenomenon and is largely confined to certain cancers arising in embryonic cells, which of course are normally programmed to disappear soon after birth). To complicate matters still further, it is also clear that fully invasive cancers can sometimes emerge after little or no preliminary warning.[14] So the only absolutely satisfactory way to judge screening programs is to compare two populations, a group of women who are regularly checked and a carefully matched control group. The results of such comparisons are discussed later in the chapter.

Other forms of cancer often seem to develop where there is some visibly abnormal, potentially precancerous condition. For all of these, too, the precursor conditions are much more common

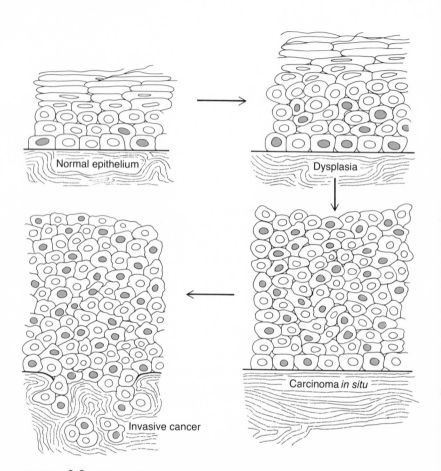

FIGURE 9-3   The evolution of cancer of the cervix. The program of cell renewal in cervical epithelium can be demonstrated by incubating a piece of the epithelium in the presence of a radioactive precursor of DNA (e.g., tritiated thymidine); cells that are about to divide will become labeled (shown here as having black nuclei), making it possible to see how strictly any section of epithelium is obeying the normal rules of cell replacement. *Normal epithelium* is regularly arranged, and cell division is confined almost entirely to the basal layer. In *dysplasia* some loss of regularity occurs, and cell division is seen at some distance from the basal layer. In *carcinoma in situ,* little order remains, cell division occurs at every level and hardly any differentiation is occurring. Finally, in an *invasive cancer* the cells have spread through the basement membrane into the underlying tissues.

than the corresponding cancers. For example, the conventional estimate for the incidence of cancer of the prostate in 70-year-old men is about 200 cases per 100,000 men per year, or 0.2%; but routine autopsies of 70-year-old men who had died of other causes have shown microscopic invasive cancers in 15 to 20%.[15] Similarly, in areas of the world like Australia and the southern United States, most men over the age of 65 show skin lesions that are thought to be precancerous, although only a minority of these lesions actually progress to form cancers.[16]

To return to cancer of the cervix, some idea of the underlying nature of these progressive abnormalities comes from cell-lineage studies in X-chromosome mosaics (see p. 18). The normal cervical epithelium, like any other part of the body, is made up of a multitude of small families of cells that do not appear to be in competition with each other; in other words, it is like a fine mosaic, where no one piece is infringing on the territory of its neighbors. However, even in the milder form of abnormality called dysplasia we find that the fine mosaicism of the epithelium has been lost, and the whole area has been taken over by a single family of cells.[17] It seems therefore that one of the earliest steps in the sequence leading to a cancer is the emergence of families that are able to displace their neighbors. No doubt this is partly the result of some intrinsic change in the cells (e.g., mutation) that enables them to compete for territory, but the whole process will presumably be accelerated by anything that causes cell death and so creates an opportunity for competition to occur; the situation is somewhat analogous to a tropical forest, which retains a nice balance of different species of trees until it is deliberately defoliated, at which point the rules of the competition are suddenly changed and the forest is overrun by bamboo. As time passes, further variants are likely to emerge within the first expanding family of cells so that cellular aggression gradually but constantly increases, ending with the formation of an invasive cancer.

Described in these terms, the evolution of a cancer can be viewed as the operation of Darwinian selection among competing populations of dividing cells. In fact, as mentioned in an earlier chapter, the surprising feature is that the tissues of the body normally preserve their initial fine mosaicism right into old age, indicating that usually there can be little or no competition between adjacent cells.

The early appearance of expanding families of cells during the evolution of cancers must have an important effect on the exact way variant cells accumulate with time. As pointed out in Chapter 4, the exact number of steps required to create a cancer could be determined from the relationship between age and incidence, provided that all steps occurred at the same, unchanging rate. If, however, the first step gives the altered cell a survival advantage so that it can steadily increase in number at the expense of normal cells, there will be a corresponding steady increase in the chance that somewhere there is a cell undergoing the next step, simply because as time goes on the size of the families of cells that have taken the first step steadily increases. We should therefore expect to find that the carcinogens which act early in the sequence are those producing variant cells capable of competing successfully against their neighbors, whereas later in the sequence of events the most powerful carcinogens may be those that stimulate competition. Obviously we must learn more about the forces that prevent competition if we are to understand the successive steps of carcinogenesis and know what kinds of agent are likely to be responsible.

The Later Stages of Human Cancer. Death or Recovery

Understanding the early steps in carcinogenesis is important for prevention. But the fate of each patient will depend on whether the cancer has already undergone metastasis at the time of diagnosis. If it has spread beyond the reach of local surgery some more general treatment such as radiotherapy or chemotherapy will be necessary.

It is not the object of this book to discuss the particularities of the different treatments of cancer. Nevertheless, some estimate must be made of the overall effectiveness of the various treatments because (apart from any possible preventive measures) it is on these terms that cancer research must finally be judged.

The results of treatment vary greatly from one class of cancer to another. For example, the commoner varieties of skin cancer are easily treated, seldom undergo metastasis, and are not a significant cause of mortality. In contrast the commonest kind of lung cancer is somewhat inaccessible to surgery, spreads rapidly, and usually causes death within a few months of diagnosis. Other cancers lie somewhere between these extremes in terms of the likelihood of permanent cure and the average number of years remaining for patients who are not cured. The usual way of summarizing the results of treatment is to give, for each type of cancer, the percentage of patients who are still alive five years after diagnosis of the cancer. But close scrutiny reveals that this statistic may be very misleading. For example, simply advancing the time of diagnosis by a year will automatically increase the proportion of patients surviving five years after diagnosis, even if the natural course of the disease and the time of death are totally unchanged; furthermore, any screening program will tend to detect cases that might otherwise have been missed (i.e., that are not so malignant), and this too will increase the average survival rate of diagnosed cases.

There is, however, a much simpler way of judging whether there have been any major advances that significantly affect the death rate from cancer.[18] People who do not have cancer worry about cancer as a whole; they want to know what is the chance that they will die of cancer in any particular year of their life, and this is a question that we can easily answer. From this point of view, there has been no recent, major advance. The chance of dying of cancer has not altered greatly in the United States in the past 35 years.[19] For white males, the total mortality from nonrespiratory cancers has not changed, while deaths from lung cancer have continued to climb steadily upwards, causing the total cancer mortality in each age group to rise by about 30% (Figure 9-4). For white females, cancer mortality in each age group dropped about 15% in the 1950s (Figure 9-5). Of course these death rates do reflect a certain amount of give-and-take. Some cancers (such as cancer of the stomach and cervix) are becoming less common, and others (such as cancer of the lung and various forms of leukemia) are more common.

For some types of cancer, successful methods of chemotherapy have been developed. For example, it now seems probable that, given the proper facilities, most cases of acute lymphatic leukemia in children (about 0.2% of all cancers) and of Hodgkin's disease (about 1.0%), as well as some other very rare childhood cancers, could be cured by these treatments.[20] Unfortunately, they are not simple to apply, and that is probably why as a general rule the patients who go to private hospitals are more likely to be cured than those who are treated in the equivalent county hospitals. Certainly, these new treatments have thus far not produced any detectable decline in the total annual cancer mortality

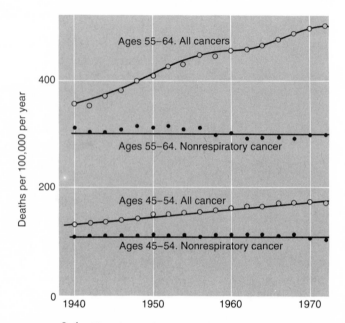

FIGURE 9-4   The change in cancer mortality for white males in the United States since 1940, shown for two different age groups. Because lung cancer is starting to contribute so much to the total (especially for males), the rate for nonrespiratory cancers is also given.

even for children—the group for which the most successes have been reported. In short, for cancer as a whole, there has been little advance. Indeed, the skin cancers aside, only about one in three of all cancer patients survive five years after diagnosis.[21]

The Results of Screening Programs

The main advances in the treatment of the common cancers came in the 1950s and were apparently due to a decrease in immediate postoperative mortality, brought about by the invention of antibiotics and better forms of anesthesia. There have not, however, been comparable improvements in the treatment of metastases. So, for most varieties of cancer, the decisive question for each patient still remains whether the cancer has been detected and excised before it has produced its first metastasis. Because there has been so little advance in the treatment of metastases, the emphasis has recently shifted to developing screening programs

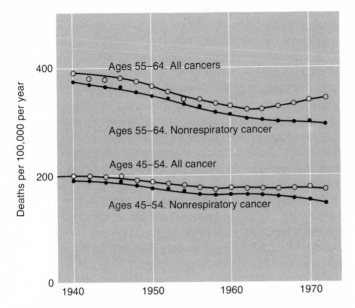

FIGURE 9-5   The change in cancer mortality for white females
in the United States since 1940, shown for two different age groups.

aimed at detecting the common cancers while they are still
localized.

Obviously, the primary cancer arises before the metastasis, and
so it follows that advancing the time of diagnosis must do some
good. But we should remember when we come to judge the various screening programs that there is no way of predicting by any
theoretical argument exactly how much good they will do. It is a
misconception to think that the natural history of every cancer
consists of growth to a size at which diagnosis becomes possible,
followed inevitably by metastasis after some constant interval of
time. Some cancers seem to be incapable of spreading to distant
sites; others produce multiple metastases while the primary
cancer is still too small to be detected. So only for a limited,
intermediate group will advancing the time of diagnosis be of any
benefit. And the proportion of patients who fall into this group
cannot be predicted but has to be determined in a properly controlled experiment.

Perhaps the best controlled experiment was a program in New
York, in which 31,000 women were checked annually for breast
cancer by all the available techniques including radiography, for
a period of 3 years, and a similar group were left as controls.[22]

The comparison was therefore the very direct one of determining whether the test group actually had fewer deaths from breast cancer than the controls. So far the tally stands at 70 deaths in the test group, and 108 in the controls—a saving of 38 lives.[23] Such a calculating, cold-blooded approach would seem to be justified when the results are examined a little more closely. It turns out that the saving occurred only in women older than 50, indicating that in younger women the breast cancers that are capable of metastasis tend to spread too early to be intercepted with the use of available technology; it seems therefore as if we are dealing with two distinct diseases, not with one. This is an important finding because it suggests that in women under the age of 50 the deaths from cancer, produced by the process of screening (which includes irradiation), would probably exceed the deaths that could be prevented. In other words, given existing technology, if screening for breast cancer is to be done at all it should be confined to women over the age of 50. That restriction is something a less well designed experiment would probably not have revealed.

In fact, the argument for proper design goes deeper than that. Once a program has been launched and has captured the public's imagination, it becomes no longer practicable or even politic to set up an experiment with proper controls. This is why it is no longer easy to gauge exactly the benefits of screening for cancer of the cervix. Although the death rate from cervical cancer can certainly be measured in the screened and the unscreened, the two groups are not properly comparable. The women most willing to be screened tend to be the better educated, and they are known to have a lower incidence of cancer of the cervix;[24] further, the analysis is complicated by the fact that the incidence is steadily falling even among those who are not being screened.[25]

Apart from the difficulty in determining their effectiveness, screening programs raise another problem. For every cancer they detect they reveal perhaps five or ten other abnormalities, many of which have the appearance of being precancerous. As long as it is impossible to tell which of these will progress to cancer they must all be treated, and this presents an economic problem. It would be beyond the resources of the United States, let alone any other country, to treat all the potentially precancerous lesions that could be detected with the limited screening procedures available today if these procedures were applied to the entire population. But prospects for the future are discussed in the remaining chapter.

PROSPECTS 10
for the FUTURE

At present, the prospects for finding a quick solution to the cancer problem seem rather slight.

For most varieties of cancer the existing methods of treatment are not very successful, and no major improvements appear to be in sight. In particular, screening programs to advance the time of diagnosis and improve the results of conventional treatment are having only limited success and are too expensive to be used on any large scale.

Prevention seems to be a feasible alternative to cure, but it will work only if the public is willing to adopt a more frugal diet and forgo certain indulgences (e.g., smoking, sunbathing, and promiscuity, to name some of the carcinogenic habits that have been identified). Whether this approach is practical remains to be seen.

The only other, long-term strategy is to seek a much more sophisticated understanding of the forces that control the cells of the body, in the hope that a really specific way of controlling cancer cells can be discovered.

The object of all cancer research is simply to stop cancer from being a major cause of death, and it is in this light that the research must ultimately be judged. In fact, the possible solutions to the cancer problem are limited to three main strategies: improving the existing methods of treatment, inventing new methods, or preventing the disease from occurring in the first place. This chapter considers the prospects for each of these in turn.

Screening Programs

Modern surgery can reach almost anywhere but it fails with cancer when the disease has started to spread to multiple distant sites scattered throughout the body. As long as there are no very successful drugs for treating metastases, the only obvious way of improving the results of surgery is to press for earlier diagnosis in the hope of catching more cases before spread has occurred.

As pointed out in the previous chapter, the gain from earlier diagnosis seems to be rather limited. Most cancers that have a strong propensity for undergoing metastasis seem to spread rather early in their history, before diagnosis is really practicable, and the maximum reduction in mortality, achievable by early diagnosis, is apparently no more than about 50% at best (for cancer of the cervix),[1] and for many cancers it can be much less.[2] There are, however, some more serious objections to putting great faith into the development of further screening programs.

First is the matter of cost. The New York breast cancer program checked 31,000 women annually for about three years, and this so far has been credited with saving the lives of 38 women, roughly one for every 2000 tests. The people who ran the program have calculated the cost of each test could conceivably be reduced to as little as $25,[3] which would lower the bill to $50,000 per life saved. At first sight this may seem a small price to pay; indeed, a good case can be made for continuing that particular program and the rather less expensive test for cancer of the cervix. But these are isolated examples. If similar procedures could be devised for all the other forms of cancer, the bill would be enormous. It works out to about $15 billion a year, if you calculate either the cost of preventing 350,000 deaths a year at the price of $50,000 each, or the cost of testing everyone in the United States over the age of 45 once a year for each of 10 varieties of cancer at the price of $25 a test. This would represent a massive increase in expenditure, because at present the total cost of treating all cancer cases in the United States is about $3.5 billion a year.[4] In fact, the calculation is for the hypothetical minimum costs of making the diagnosis and does not include the additional cost of treating all the extra, possibly precancerous conditions that would be detected in the tests. For most types of cancer, these precancerous conditions tend to outnumber the cancers by at least five to one.[5]

If screening could be confined to particular high-risk groups, the cost would be correspondingly reduced. This is possible for certain rare cancers; for example, there are several uncommon, inherited traits that are associated with an exceptionally high risk for particular cancers—e.g., retinal cancers in children inheriting the trait for retinoblastoma, colon cancers in young adults inheriting the trait for polyposis coli, skin cancers in people with xeroderma pigmentosum, and so on—and these patients have to be watched very carefully.[6] For some of the common cancers, it is already possible to identify particular groups of people with a higher than average risk (e.g., women with a family history of breast cancer, people who smoke heavily, and so on), and in time more ways will be found for identifying such groups;[7] for example, it seems that the people who have the highest risk of colon cancer may be identified in advance because their feces contain certain carcinogens and species of bacteria that are missing in most of the population.[8] There is no indication, however, that these high-risk groups for the common cancers constitute such a small proportion of the whole population that the saving in costs would be substantial. After all, about one in three people get some form of cancer at some point in their life.

The other weakness of screening programs is that the general public does not view them as very effective. So people will tend not to use them. In the absence of any artificial propaganda it seems unlikely, for example, that most women will continue to present themselves regularly for Pap smears. Cancer of the cervix causes only 5% of all deaths in women, and screening probably reduces this percentage by twofold (thereby saving fewer lives than would be saved by wearing seat belts or giving up cigarettes). To many women, especially the poor and less well educated, this reduction will probably seem too slight to warrant the expense and inconvenience of continued check-ups.

The prospects would be altered completely if some way were found for achieving much earlier diagnosis. For example, if some easily measured characteristic cell product were discovered that circulated in the blood of all cancer patients from the moment their cancer was first formed, the efficiency of screening might be greatly increased and the cost could come down. Various possible products have been suggested (e.g., the carcinoembryonic antigen produced by cancers of the colon).[9] However, with a few exceptions (such as the hormone, chorionic gonadotrophin, which is a characteristic product of the very rare cancers of the placenta),[10] they have not proved to be reliable enough because most of them are rather nonspecific and arise in other, noncancerous conditions. So far, they are therefore used more for monitoring the progress or recurrence of cancers than for making early diagnosis.

Until there is some such technological breakthrough it is hard to view screening programs as anything other than an interim measure, which could produce a slight drop in mortality and would give the impression of activity at a time when the public has been led to expect great advances.

Prevention

Because the major cancers vary greatly in incidence from one country to another, they are thought to be caused by environmental factors. Sooner or later we are bound to discover what the most important factors are, and it will then be possible to think about prevention instead of treatment. The relative emphasis we place on this endeavor depends, however, on how long we think it will take to discover the major causes and, once these have been identified, how practicable it will be to remove them from the environment.

Already the preventable causes of some cancers are known. Lung cancer is due almost entirely to smoking, and skin cancer to sunlight. Cancer of the large intestine seems to be produced by a particular combination of diet and perhaps the action of certain bacteria in the colon, and it should not be long before someone will set up a prospective experiment in active prevention by altering diet and perhaps also bacterial flora. The incidence of breast cancer is related to diet and reproductive history; so for this cancer, too, experiments in prevention are certainly conceivable. If cancer of the lung, large intestine, and breast could be prevented, that would be a fairly substantial beginning because the three together cause nearly half of all cancer deaths.

At this point the strategy encounters various difficulties.[11] Cancer of the lung is due to a pleasant and highly addictive habit; cancer of the large intestine and breast are most common in affluent countries and so are presumably associated with some desirable habit, such as a high-fat diet, that the rich nations can afford and the others cannot; other potentially harmful customs are drinking alcohol (which contributes to cancer of the esophagus) and promiscuity (which is an important causal factor in cancer of the cervix). Any attempt to prevent these cancers will require people to give up pleasurable habits, an exercise that may have only limited success in the absence of acceptable substitutes.[12] For example, the richer and better educated sector of the population are now smoking less than they used to.[13] In contrast, the smoking patterns of the poor have not changed, suggesting that the habit is more important to them; in effect, they seem to have decided (probably quite correctly) that the life of old people who are poor is not very enjoyable and that it is therefore not worth making sacrifices in one's youth in order to gain a few extra years at the far end. Furthermore, the man in the street has unfortunately been sold the idea that the "breakthrough" cure for cancer is just around the corner. So he will see little sense in taking any inconvenient steps now in order to prevent a cancer that he is not going to get for another 10 or 20 years by which time, he has been told, there should be a cure.

The other barrier to preventing lung cancer is economic. Cigarette smoking is known to cause death not only from lung cancer but also from bronchitis and heart disease, and the relationship between smoking and general ill health and mortality is well quantified. So it is possible to estimate fairly precisely what the economic consequences would be if any given percentage of the population stopped smoking. The calculation has recently been carried out for England, where health care and social security are run by the state and the costs are therefore easily assessed.[14] As one might expect, a reduction in smoking would increase the gross national product (partly by reducing absence from work and partly by saving lives and therefore increasing the population) and would decrease the amount of chronic respiratory disease and therefore the costs of health care. But what was not expected was the finding that, from the government's point of view, these gains are only temporary. Even leaving aside any consideration of revenue from the tax on tobacco, the gains would be wiped out after about 20 years by the resulting large increase in the population who are past retirement age and who therefore require social security and more than the average amount of health care but do not generate much income for the state; and from that time onwards the losses will always be greater than the gains. The sums of money are surprisingly large. The calculated saving on social security payments and health care, that the cigarette brings because it diminishes the number of old people, is enough to pay many times over for all government sponsored medical research. In addition, the revenue from the tax on tobacco is almost enough to pay for all the salaries and running costs for all the hospitals in England. Faced with such financial considerations, most governments do not seem benevolent enough to forgo revenue in order to support preventive medicine. Their actions would suggest they have decided the only practical solution is to encourage the design of a cigarette that is safer but is still addictive and still contains some unique taxable ingredient. The production of low-tar cigarettes is a step in that direction, although so far the new cigarettes still seem to pose some risk, though not as much as the old ones.[15]

Whether every major attempt at cancer prevention is going to encounter such difficult economic problems will not be known until the other important carcinogens in our environment have been identified. But with any luck, they may be identified fairly soon. In the past few years several rapid, inexpensive tests for carcinogenicity have been devised, in which bacteria or bacterial viruses are used as the test organisms, and these new methods probably give just as accurate a prediction as any test on experimental animals (see p. 104). It is now at least conceivable that the important carcinogens in our environment could be determined simply by identifying which substances are present in the human body that are capable of causing mutations in bacteria, and then tracing these substances back to their source. For example, in the absence of any epidemiology, it would have been possible, solely by testing for bacterial mutagenicity, to single out smoking as a likely major cause of cancer, because tobacco tars have been shown to be highly mutagenic and the main group of people with measurable levels of mutagens in their urine are the people who smoke.[16]

So far, these tests for bacterial mutagenicity have been applied mainly to screening the many unnatural substances to which we are exposed—the synthetic dyes, pesticides, and preservatives on which our modern way of life seems to depend. Despite a lot of publicity there is little evidence that the chemical industry causes much of the current total cancer incidence. As pointed out in Chapter 4, with the exception of lung cancer, none of the common cancers are much commoner now than they were 50 years ago, whereas most of the chemicals people are worried about were introduced only after World War II. In fact it seems more likely that the main determinant of cancer is diet rather than industry, and that we should be looking for mutagens (or perhaps promoters) that are formed in the body from the normal ingredients in our diet.

Although industry does not seem to be responsible for any of the common cancers, a good argument can nevertheless be made for checking carefully all new materials released for human consumption. Most of the artificial reactive chemicals in our environment are of very recent origin; for example the annual consumption of pesticides, synthetic rubber, and plastics in the United States has risen more than 100-fold since 1950. So it may be still too soon to see if any of them affect cancer incidence. The answer, of course, is for the chemical manufacturers to test each new compound for mutagenicity before they have made a large investment and become reluctant to stop production. It is conceivable therefore that the rapid, inexpensive ways of testing for mutagenicity (and probable carcinogenicity) have been invented just in time.

In summary, modern methods of testing should enable us to prevent new forms of cancer arising as a result of further advances in industrial technology. It is also conceivable that the preventable causes of the common cancers will soon be identified. What remains to be determined, however, is the public response to programs of prevention. People may not be willing to change their life style in order to diminish their chance of getting cancer in old age. Nor is it certain that they should be frightened, legislated, or otherwise coerced into doing so.

Treatment

For most forms of cancer, excision of the primary tumor results in an immediate improvement in the quality of the patient's life; in addition several other methods of treatment, such as irradiation and chemotherapy, can reduce the extent of a cancer, bring some relief from the symptoms and prolong the patient's life. Despite indubitable advances in the treatment of some cancers, such as Hodgkin's disease and certain forms of leukemia which can now often be cured by chemotherapy, the fact remains that only about one-third of all cancer patients survive for more than 5 years from the time of diagnosis. Therefore, taken as a whole, the available methods of treatment are plainly not very successful.

The public has been led to expect more than this. We live in an age of scientific accomplishment, in which we conquer the great pestilences, harness the atom, and send a man to the moon and back. So it has become all too easy to imagine that everything we desire must automatically lie within the compass of our technology. As a result, the conquest of cancer has come to be regarded much as if it were some five-year plan on a collective farm, which is certain to succeed provided everyone has enough enthusiasm.

To estimate the prospects for discovering an efficient cure for cancer, it is worth considering how some of the other triumphs of applied biology came to pass, for we can learn something from their history. The various revolutions in agriculture were part of a gradual progression, occurring in the course of millennia, and the recent contributions of science to agriculture have really only accelerated the progress rather than initiated something completely new; for example, selective breeding had been conducted for thousands of years before the geneticist systematized the rules of inheritance, and the practice of rotating crops was established some time before much was known about plant nutrition. Similarly, the battle against infectious diseases has been waged, for the most part, with the use of well established methods: the main advance, in terms of numbers of lives saved (see p. 7), was probably a by-product of the improvement of nutrition and hygiene that had been made in the 19th century; the practice of preventing the spread of diseases by isolating the patients dates back to the leper colonies of the middle ages; today's vaccines, which have virtually eradicated diseases like smallpox, are descended from customs dating back to ancient Egypt; indeed only since the 1930s has science provided really innovative means of curing infections, with the discovery of antibiotics and pesticides. These are so successful, however, that they have set the standard. To the lay public the conquest of cancer means nothing less than the discovery of some agent as effective as one of the standard antibiotics. In order to estimate how long we must wait for that kind of cure it is worth considering what makes the antibiotics so successful.

Penicillin is a typical antibiotic. It is produced by a fungus and kills certain species of bacteria because it is chemically very similar to one of the components built into the bacterial surface, and it therefore blocks one of the enzymes involved in synthesis of the surface and stops the bacteria from growing. Other antibiotics like streptomycin block the machinery in bacteria for translating nucleic acids into proteins; others like the sulfonamides block particular steps in bacterial metabolism; and so on. The success of all these antibiotics hinges on the crucial fact that bacterial and mammalian chemistries are somewhat different. We may speak the same basic language as bacteria—i.e., use exactly the same genetic code (see Chapter 6)—but we have gone our separate ways for over a billion years and this divergence has left its mark at many points. It is possible therefore to find substances that are poisonous for mammalian cells but not for bacteria (e.g., the toxins formed by diphtheria and cholera); or that are poisonous for bacteria but not for mammalian cells, and these are the antibiotics.

Thus the antibacterial antibiotics are not the right model. Because the cancer cell will necessarily have the same underlying chemistry as the normal cells of the body, it is obviously going to be much harder to find a drug that is lethal specifically for cancer. Certainly, whenever a special way has been found for killing some particular class of cell (e.g., killing thyroid cells by administering radioactive iodine, which is then used by the cells to make the iodine-containing hormone, thyroxin), the method usually proves to be incapable of distinguishing between cancer cells and normal cells.

However, some special signalling systems must be controlling the extent of cell multiplication in each tissue, and it is conceivable that these could be used at least for controlling the growth of a cancer. For example, tissue such as skin epithelium has a strictly local function, that of covering every part of our surface, so that the signals controlling the multiplication of skin cells must be strictly localized; but, for organs like liver or bone marrow, which have a general function, some process for monitoring the total quantity of tissue and some general control of cell division must be operating. Sooner or later, these tissue-specific signals will be identified. Like the bacteria-specific chemical reactions that are vulnerable to antibiotics, these signals may eventually be made the target of attack by some tissue-specific form of chemotherapy.

So far, the best understood signals are the hormones produced by the endocrine glands (such as the thyroid, adrenals, pituitary, and ovaries), and some of these can be used to help in the control of certain cancers. For example, the multiplication of breast epithelium is under the overall control of ovarian hormones (such as the estrogens) and breast cancer is sometimes treated by removing the source of these hormones; conversely, raising the level of estrogens in a male is sometimes used to suppress cancers of the prostate. These treatments, however, are not completely specific for the target cells and they are often accompanied by undesirable side effects; furthermore, even the most susceptible cancers tend eventually to become resistant to hormone therapy.

One other completely different method might be used to control cancer. The function of the immune system is to produce antibodies and killer cells directed specifically against particular targets (antigens) that are foreign to the body. Although apparently this system does not normally attack cancer cells (see p. 140), it could possibly be provoked into doing so, especially as cancer cells are known frequently to bear novel surface antigens that mark them as unusual if not actually foreign. A recent development in cancer therapy has been the attempt to stimulate the immune system by injecting large quantities of some very powerful antigen (e.g., killed diphtheria bacilli, or the attenuated strain of tuberculosis that is used as a vaccine). The results of such treatments have to be judged by comparing the survival rate of treated patients with that of matched controls; whether any of the procedures are effective is still unresolved. However, even if these crude methods turn out to be worthless, the possibility remains that some way of harnessing the immune system will eventually be found.

In the absence of any marked success with these logical ways of attacking cancer cells, the only remaining strategy has been to embark on a systematic investigation of all the agents known to kill mammalian cells, in the hope of finding some that are more lethal to cancers than to normal tissues. Surprisingly, this rather forlorn exercise has already produced a certain number of notable successes. Some forms of skin cancer respond very well to X-irradiation, and several quite rare cancers affecting cells of the immune system (e.g., Hodgkin's disease, and one kind of acute leukemia) can now apparently be cured by combined techniques of radiotherapy and chemotherapy, in a fairly high proportion of cases. Even where cure proves impossible, such treatments, administered in moderation, can alleviate symptoms and prolong life. All the drugs, however, are very toxic and can produce most unpleasant side effects, and in using them, medical practitioners have sometimes acquired the reputation of battling more strongly for their patients' survival than the patients themselves would wish.

Viewed overall, these nonsurgical methods have not had a major impact on cancer mortality as a whole. Furthermore, much of the chemotherapy practiced today must be accompanied by elaborate hospital care and is therefore very expensive; in this respect it is reminiscent of some of the complicated and largely unsuccessful treatments for infections such as tuberculosis, typhoid, and pneumonia that were used before the advent of the much cheaper and more effective treatment with antibiotics. Nevertheless, doctors who treat patients in the large cancer centers believe they will gradually find better and better combinations of drugs for treating more and more types of cancer and, in this way, will eventually start to make major inroads into cancer mortality, without having to understand very much about the mechanism underlying the origin and spread of the disease.

Thus far, however, there is no treatment for any of the major lethal cancers that is as effective as the antibiotics. Like many others,[17] I find it hard to visualize the discovery of such a treatment until much more has been learned about the normal control of cell growth in the intact animal. Indeed, the very prospect seems so remote that it does not even enter into the speculative, day-to-day conversation of people engaged in cancer research; at present so little is known about the control of cell growth that there is no way of guessing when we will arrive at the necessary understanding—it could be in the next 10 or 20 years, or not for another century.

REFERENCES

Note: As far as possible the references given in this list are taken from readily accessible sources, such as the major scientific journals. In addition the following books on cancer and ongoing series of reviews of cancer research treat in much greater detail most of the subjects mentioned in the preceding chapters.

(a) *Cancer,* Volumes 1–6. R. W. Raven, ed. Butterworth & Co., London (1957–1960).

(b) *Cancer: A Comprehensive Treatise,* Volumes 1–4. F. F. Becker, ed. Plenum Press, New York and London (1975).

(c) *Advances in Cancer Research.* Volumes 1–. Academic Press, New York (1953–).

(d) *Progress in Experimental Tumor Research,* Volumes 1–. S. Karger, Basel and New York (1960–).

(e) National Cancer Institute Monographs. U.S. Government Printing Office, Washington, D.C., (1959–).

CHAPTER 2

1. A collection of articles on the changes in growth rate of the human population in the course of the past few thousand years appeared in *Scientific American*, September 1974.

2. T. McKeown, R. G. Brown, and R. G. Record. "An interpretation of the modern rise of population in Europe." *Popul. Stud.* **26**, 345–382 (1972).

3. The Registrar General's *Statistical Review of England and Wales* for the year 1972. Part I. *Tables, Medical.* H. M. Stationary Office, London.

4. The various consequences of the impending change in age distribution of the United States population are discussed in *Population and the American Future*, U.S. Government Printing Office, No. 5258-0002, Washington, D.C.

CHAPTER 3

1. The total number of cells in the body and their rate of production in adult life have been determined rather precisely for the rat. The numbers given here are based on the assumption that we have about 200 times as many cells as a rat. See M. Enesco and C. P. Leblond. "Increase in cell number as a factor in the growth of the organs and tissues of the young male rat." *J. Embryol. Exp. Morph.* **10**, 530–562 (1962).

2. C. P. Leblond. "Classification of cell populations on the basis of their proliferative behavior." *Natn. Cancer Inst. Monogr.* **14**, 119–150 (1964).

3. P. J. Fialkow. "The origin and development of human tumors studied with cell markers." *New Engl. J. Med.* **291**, 26–35 (1974).
P. J. Fialkow. "Clonal origin of human tumors." *Biochim. Biophys. Acta* **458**, 283–321 (1976).

4. M. N. Nesbitt. "X chromosome inactivation mosaicism in the mouse." *Devl. Biol.* **26**, 252–263 (1971).
N. Takagi. "Differentiation of X chromosomes in early female mouse embryos." *Expl. Cell. Res.* **86**, 127–135 (1974).
Editorial. "Number of cells at the time of X inactivation." *Nature* **249**, 9–11 (1974).

5. S. M. Gartler, E. Gandini, H. T. Hutchison, B. Campbell, and G. Zechhi. "Glucose-6-phosphate dehydrogenase mosaicism: utilization in the study of hair follicle variegation." *Ann. Hum. Genet.* **35**, 1–7 (1971).

N. Feder. "Solitary cells and enzyme exchange in tetraparental mice." *Nature* **263**, 67–69 (1976).

6. P. J. Fialkow. *New Engl. J. Med.* **291** (1974); Fialkow, *Biochim. Biophys. Acta* **458** (1976).

7. P. C. Nowell and D. A. Hungerford. "A minute chromosome in human chronic granulocytic leukemia." *Science* **132**, 1497 (1960).

8. C. R. Dorn, D. O. N. Taylor, F. L. Frye, H. H. Hibbard. "Survey of animal neoplasms in Alameda and Contra Costa counties, California. 1. Methodology and description of cases." *J. Natn. Cancer Inst.* **40**, 295–305 (1968).
W. A. Priester, N. Mantel. "Occurrence of tumors in domestic animals. Data from 12 United States and Canadian colleges of veterinary medicine." *J. Natn. Cancer Inst.* **47**, 1333–1344 (1971).

9. International Union against Cancer. *Illustrated tumor nomenclature.* Springer-Verlag, Berlin (1965).

10. W. Montagna and W. C. Lobitz. *The Epidermis.* Academic Press, New York (1964).

11. O. H. Iversen, R. Bjerknes and F. Devik. "Kinetics of cell renewal, cell migration and cell loss in the hairless mouse dorsal epidermis." *Cell Tissue Kinet.* **1**, 351–367 (1968).
C. S. Potten. "The epidermal proliferative unit: the possible role of the central basal cell." *Cell and Tissue Kinet.* **7**, 77–88 (1974).
I. C. Mackenzie. "Spatial distribution of mitosis in mouse epidermis." *Anat. Rec.* **181**, 705–710 (1975).

12. S. Rothberg, R. G. Crounse, and J. L. Lee. "Glycine-C^{14} incorporation into the proteins of normal stratum corneum and the abnormal stratum corneum of psoriasis." *J. Invest. Derm.* **37**, 497–505 (1961).

13. E. J. Van Scott and R. P. Reinertson. "The modulating influence of stromal environment on epithelial cells studied in human autotransplants." *J. Invest. Derm.* **36**, 109–117 (1961).
R. J. Goss. *Regulation of organ and tissue growth.* Academic Press, New York (1972).
R. H. Sawyer, U. K. Abbott, and J. D. Trelford. "Inductive interactions between human dermis and chick chorionic epithelium." *Science* **175**, 527–529 (1972).

14. T. Gibson and W. Norris. "Skin fragments removed by injection needles." *Lancet* **ii**, 983–985 (1958).

15. J. D. Ebert and I. M. Sussex. *Interacting Systems in Development.* Holt, Rinehart, and Winston, Inc., New York (1970).

16. E. J. Van Scott and T. M. Ekel. "Kinetics of hyperplasia in psoriasis." *Archs. Derm.* **88**, 373–381 (1963).

17. E. J. Van Scott. "Reaction patterns of normal and neoplastic epithelium." *Adv. Biol. Skin* **7**, 75–87 (1965).

18. F. Urbach, R. E. Davies, and P. D. Forbes. "Ultraviolet radiation and skin cancer in man." *Adv. Biol. Skin.* **7**, 195–214 (1965).

19. General descriptions of the common cancers are given in all the standard textbooks of pathology.

20. V. C. Twitty and M. C. Niu. "The motivation of cell migration, studied by isolation of embryonic pigment cells singly and in small groups *in vitro.*" *J. Exp. Zool.* **125**, 541–573 (1954).
    J. P. Trinkaus. *Cells into Organs. The Forces That Shape the Embryo.* Prentice-Hall, Englewood Cliffs, New Jersey (1969).

21. L. J. Faulkin and K. B. Deome. "Regulation of growth and spacing of gland elements in the mammary fat pad of the C3H mouse." *J. Natn. Cancer Inst.* **24**, 953–969 (1960).
    L. J. Faulkin. "Hyperplastic lesions of mouse mammary glands after treatment with 3-methylcholanthrene." *J. Natn. Cancer Inst.* **36**, 289–297 (1966).

22. K. Kratochwil and P. Schwartz. "Tissue interaction in androgen response of embryonic mammary rudiment of mouse: identification of target tissue for testosterone." *Proc. Natn. Acad. Sci. U.S.A.* **73**, 4041–4044 (1976).

23. R. E. Billingham and W. K. Silvers. "Studies on the conservation of epidermal specificities of skin and certain mucosas in adult mammals." *J. Exp. Med.* **125**, 429–446 (1967).

CHAPTER 4

1. R. Doll. *Prevention of Cancer. Pointers from Epidemiology.*" The Nuffield Provincial Hospitals Trust, London (1967).
   J. Higginson. "Present trends in cancer epidemiology." *Canad. Cancer Conference* **8**, 40–75 (1969).

2. For a general review of the history of cancer epidemiology, see J. Clemmesen, "Statistical studies in malignant neoplasms," *Acta. Path. Microbiol. Scand. Suppl.* **174** (1965).
   For more recent statistics, see A. M. Lilienfeld, M. L. Levin, and I. I. Kessler, *Cancer in the United States*, Harvard University Press, Cambridge, Mass. (1972)
   J. F. Fraumeni. *Persons at High Risk of Cancer.* Academic Press, New York (1975).

3. J. C. Fisher and J. H. Hollomon. "A hypothesis for the origin of cancer foci." *Cancer* **4**, 916–918 (1951).
   C. O. Nordling. "A new theory on the cancer-inducing mechanism." *Brit. J. Cancer* **7**, 68–72 (1953).

P. Armitage and R. Doll. "The age distribution of cancer and a multi-stage theory of carcinogenesis." *Brit. J. Cancer* **8**, 1–12 (1954).
J. C. Fisher. "Multiple-mutation theory of carcinogenesis." *Nature* **181**, 651–652 (1958).

4. Of course, if an early stage in the sequence of steps produces a locally expanding population of cells, the number of cells at risk for subsequent steps could rise steeply with time and the number steps required to make a cancer might be fewer than the simple model would suggest; see P. Armitage and R. Doll, "A two-stage theory of carcinogenesis in relation to the age distribution of human cancer," *Brit. J. Cancer* **11**, 161–169 (1957).

5. G. S. Watson. "Age incidence curves for cancer." *Proc. Natn. Acad. Sci. U.S.A.* **74**, 1341–1342 (1977).

6. F. M. Burnet. *Immunology, Aging and Cancer. Medical Aspects of Mutation and Selection.* W. H. Freeman and Company. San Francisco (1976).

7. G. C. Williams. "Pleiotropy, natural selection, and the evolution of senescence." *Evolution.* **11**, 398–411 (1957).
W. D. Hamilton, "The moulding of senescence by natural selection." *J. Theoret. Biol.* **12**, 12–45 (1966).

8. A. Sommer and W. H. Mosley. "East Bengal cyclone of November, 1970." *Lancet* **i**, 1029–1036 (1972).

9. F. Verzar. "The aging of collagen." *Scientific American,* April (1963).

10. C. R. Hamlin and R. R. Kohn. "Determination of human chronological age by study of a collagen sample." *Exp. Gerontol.* **7**, 377–379 (1972).

11. E. P. Benditt and J. M. Benditt. "Evidence for a monoclonal origin of human atherosclerotic plaques." *Proc. Natn. Acad. Sci. U.S.A.* **70**, 1753–1756 (1973).

12. R. E. Albert, M. Vanderlaan, F. J. Burns, and M. Nishizumi. "Effect of carcinogens on chicken atherosclerosis." *Cancer Res.* **37**, 2232–2235 (1977).

13. "With regard to cancer, it is not only necessary to observe the effects of climate and local situation, but to extend our views to different employments, as those in various metals and manufactures; in mines and collieries; in the army and navy; in those who lead sedentary or active lives; in the married or single; in the different sexes, and many other circumstances. Should it be proved that women are more subject to cancer than men, we may then inquire whether married women are more liable to have the uterus or breasts affected: those who have suckled, or those who did not; and the same observations may be made of the single." The Society for Investigating the Nature and Cure of Cancer (Edinburgh, 1806), quoted by J. Clemmesen, *Acta. Path. Microbiol. Scand. Suppl.* **174** (1965).

14. International Union against Cancer. *Cancer Incidence in Five Continents*. Volume I (1966), Volume II (1970), Volume III (1977). Springer-Verlag, Berlin.

15. R. W. Miller. "Interim report: UICC international study of childhood cancer." *Int. J. Cancer* **10**, 675–677 (1972).

16. J. Higginson. "Present trends in cancer epidemiology." *Canad. Cancer Conference* **8**, 40–75 (1969).

17. A. M. Lilienfeld, M. L. Levin, and I. I. Kessler. *Cancer in the United States*. Harvard University Press, Cambridge, Mass. (1972).

18. T. Gordon, M. Crittenden and W. Haenszel. "Cancer mortality trends in the United States, 1930–1955." *Natn. Cancer Inst. Monograph* **6**, 131–350 (1961).
    F. Burbank. "Patterns in cancer mortality in the United States: 1950–1967." *Natn. Cancer Inst. Monograph* **33** (1971).

19. D. P. Burkitt. "Epidemiology of cancer of the colon and rectum." *Cancer* **28** 3–13 (1971).
    M. J. Hill, et al. "Faecal bile-acids and Clostridia in patients with cancer of the large bowel." *Lancet* **i**, 535–539 (1975).

20. H. Ingleby and J. Gershon-Cohen. "Adenosis of the female breast." *Surg. Gyn. Obst.* **99**, 199–206 (1954).
    A. T. Sandison. "An autopsy study of the adult human breast." *Natn. Cancer Inst. Monogr.* **8** (1962).
    J. R. W. Masters, J. O. Drife and J. J. Scarisbrick. "Cyclic variation of DNA synthesis in human breast epithelium." *J. Natn. Cancer Inst.* **58**, 1263–1265 (1977).

21. W. Haenszel, M. Kurihara, M. Segi, and R. K. C. Lee. "Stomach cancer among Japanese in Hawaii." *J. Natn. Cancer Inst.* **49**, 969–988 (1972).
    W. Haenszel, et al. "Large-bowel cancer in Hawaiian Japanese." *J. Natn. Cancer Inst.* **51**, 1765–1779 (1973).

22. The production of the various inbred strains of mice with high incidence of cancer is reviewed by L. Gross in his book, *Oncogenic Viruses*, Pergamon Press, Oxford (1970).

23. J. Clemmesen. "Statistical studies in malignant neoplasms." *Acta Path. Microbiol. Scand. Suppl.* **174** (1965).

24. M. T. Macklin. "Comparison of the number of breast-cancer deaths observed in relatives of breast-cancer patients, and the number expected on the basis of mortality rates." *J. Natn. Cancer Inst.* **22**, 927–951 (1959).

25. One possible exception may be the very rare inherited disease called Bloom's syndrome, in which the chromosomes of every cell undergo an abnormal number of exchanges at each division. Patients with

this condition show a raised incidence of leukemia in childhood and of stomach and large intestine cancer when they are young adults. See J. German. "Bloom's syndrome. II. The prototype of genetic disorders predisposing to chromosome instability and cancer." In J. German, ed., *Chromosomes and Cancer*, Wiley, London (1974).

26. B. S. Schoenberg. "Multiple primary malignant neoplasms: The Connecticut experience, 1935–1964." *Recent Results in Cancer Research* **58** (1977).

27. B. Harvald and M. Hauge. "Heredity of cancer elucidated by a study of unselected twins." *J. Amer. Med. Assoc.* **186,** 749–753 (1963).
R. H. Osborne and F. V. de George. "Neoplastic diseases in twins: evidence for pre- or peri-natal factors conditioning cancer susceptibility." *Cancer* **17,** 1149–1154 (1964).

28. F. Burbank. "Patterns in cancer mortality in the United States: 1950–1967." *Natn. Cancer Inst. Monograph* **33** (1971).

29. G. Kellermann, C. R. Shaw and M. Luyten-Kellermann. "Aryl hydrocarbon hydroxylase inducibility and bronchogenic carcinoma." *New Engl. J. Med.* **289,** 971–973 (1973).
A. E. H. Emery et al. Aryl-hydrocarbon-hydroxylase inducibility in patients with cancer. *Lancet* **i,** 470–472 (1978).

30. B. Paigen, et al. "Distribution of aryl hydrocarbon hydroxylase inducibility in cultured human lymphocytes." *Cancer Res.* **37,** 1829–1837 (1977).

31. For a general review of these inherited diseases, see J. German, ed., *Chromosomes and Cancer*, Wiley, London (1974).

32. P. Pott. "Chirurgical observations relative to the cataract, the polypus of the nose, the cancer of the scrotum, the different kinds of ruptures, and the mortification of the toes and feet" (1775). A facsimile of the relevant section of this remarkable work is present in the *National Cancer Institute Monograph* **10,** 7–13 (1963).

33. M. H. C. Williams. "Occupational tumours of the bladder." R. W. Raven, ed., *Cancer*, Volume III, Butterworth (1958).

34. I. J. Selikoff, E. C. Hammond, and J. Churg. "Asbestos exposure, smoking, and neoplasia." *J. Am. Med. Assn.* **204,** 106–112 (1968).
G. Berry, M. L. Newhouse, and M. Turok. "Combined effect of asbestos exposure and smoking on mortality from lung cancer in factory workers." *Lancet* **ii,** 476–479 (1972).

35. M. Essex, et al. "Horizontal transmission of feline leukemia virus under natural conditions in a feline leukemia cluster household." *Int. J. Cancer* **19,** 90–96 (1977).

36. W. S. Bailey. "Parasites and cancer: sarcoma in dogs associated with *Spirocerca lupi*." *Ann. N.Y. Acad. Sci.* **108,** 890–923 (1963).

37. W. T. Weber, P. C. Nowell and W. C. D. Hare. "Chromosome studies of a transplanted and a primary canine venereal sarcoma." *J. Natn. Cancer Inst.* **35**, 537–548 (1965).
   D. Cohen. "The biological behaviour of the transmissible venereal tumour in immunosuppressed dogs." *Eur. J. Cancer* **9**, 253–258 (1973).
38. K. Nazerian. "Marek's disease: a neoplastic disease of chickens caused by a herpesvirus." *Adv. Cancer Res.* **17**, 279–315 (1973).
39. J. Clemmesen, *Acta Path. Microbiol. Scand. Suppl.* **174** (1965).
40. I. I. Kessler. "Venereal factors in human cervical cancer. Evidence from marital clusters." *Cancer* **39**, 1912–1919 (1977).
41. L. Aurelian, B. Schumann, R. L. Marcus, and H. J. Davis. "Antibody to HSV-2 induced tumor specific antigens in serums from patients with cervical carcinoma." *Science* **181**, 161–164 (1973).
42. N. J. Vianna, et al. "Hodgkin's disease: cases with features of a community outbreak." *Ann. Intern. Med.* **77**, 169–180 (1972).
43. S. Grufferman. "Clustering and aggregation of exposures in Hodgkin's disease." *Cancer* **39**, 1829–1833 (1977).
44. R. H. Kimberlin, ed. *Slow Virus Diseases of Animals and Man.* North-Holland, Amsterdam (1976).
45. G. Manolov and Y. Manolova. "A marker band in one chromosome No. 14 in Burkitt lymphomas." *Hereditas* **69**, 300 (1971).
46. D. P. Burkitt. "Etiology of Burkitt's lymphoma—an alternative hypothesis to a vectored virus." *J. Natn. Cancer Inst.* **42**, 19–28 (1969).
   H. zur Hausen. "Biochemical approaches to detection of Epstein-Barr virus in human tumors." *Cancer Res.* **36**, 678–680 (1976).
47. R. H. Morrow, A. Kisuule, M. C. Pike and P. G. Smith. "Burkitt's lymphoma in the Mengo districts of Uganda: epidemiological features and their relationship to malaria." *J. Natn. Cancer Inst.* **56**, 479–483 (1976).

CHAPTER 5

1. R. A. Willis. "The Experimental production of tumours" (Chapter 4). *Pathology of Tumours.* Butterworths, London (1960).
2. M. B. Shimkin. "M. A. Novinsky: a note on the history of transplantation of tumours." *Cancer* **8**, 652–655 (1955).
3. K. Yamagiwa and K. Ichikawa. "Experimental study of the pathogenesis of carcinoma." *J. Cancer Res.* **3**, 1–29 (1918).
4. L. Gross. *Oncogenic Viruses.* Chapter 8. Pergamon Press, Oxford (1970).

5. Theodore Boveri. "On the problem of the origin of malignant tumors." Reprinted in J. German, ed., *Chromosomes and Cancer*. Wiley, New York (1974).

6. E. L. Kennaway. "Further experiments on cancer-producing substances." *Biochem J.* **24**, 497–504 (1930).

7. M. Blumer. "Polycyclic aromatic compounds in nature." *Scientific American*, March 1976.

8. E. Boyland. "Chemical carcinogenesis and experimental chemotherapy of cancer." *Yale J. Biol. Med.* **20**, 321–341 (1947).

CHAPTER 6

1. There are many admirable reviews of the subject of molecular genetics. See *The Molecular Basis of Life. Readings from Scientific American*, with introductions by R. H. Haynes and P. C. Hanawalt. W. H. Freeman and Company, San Francisco (1968).
J. D. Watson. *Molecular Biology of the Gene*. Benjamin, New York (1970).
G. S. Stent. *Molecular Genetics: An Introductory Narrative*. W. H. Freeman and Company, San Francisco (1971).

2. For further reading, see J. W. Drake, *The Molecular Basis of Mutation*, Holden-Day, San Francisco (1970).
A. Hollaender, ed. *Chemical Mutagens: Principles and Methods for Their Detection*. Plenum Press, New York (1971).
J. W. Drake and R. H. Baltz. "The biochemistry of mutagenesis." *Ann. Rev. Biochem.* **45**, 11–37 (1976).

3. P. Nevers and H. Saedler. "Transposable genetic elements as agents of gene instability and chromosomal rearrangements." *Nature* **268**, 109–115 (1977).

4. L. E. Orgel. "Ageing of clones of mammalian cells." *Nature* **243**, 441–445 (1973).

CHAPTER 7

1. W. F. Friedewald and P. Rous. "The initiating and promoting elements in tumor production." *J. Exp. Med.* **80**, 101–126 (1944).

2. I. Berenblum. *Carcinogenesis as a Biological Problem*. North-Holland, Oxford (1974).

3. P. Brookes and P. D. Lawley. "Evidence for the binding of polynuclear aromatic hydrocarbons to the nucleic acids of mouse skin: rela-

tion between carcinogenic power of hydrocarbons and their binding to deoxyribonucleic acid." *Nature* **202**, 781–784 (1964).

4. I. Berenblum and P. Shubik. "The role of croton oil applications, associated with a single painting of a carcinogen, in tumour induction of the mouse's skin." *Brit. J. Cancer* **1**, 379–382 (1947).
   I. Berenblum and P. Shubik. " The persistence of latent tumour cells induced in the mouse's skin by a single application of 9:10-dimethyl-1:2-benzanthracene." *Brit. J. Cancer* **3**, 384–386 (1949).

5. I. Mackenzie and P. Rous. "The experimental disclosure of latent neoplastic changes in tarred skin." *J. Exp. Med.* **73**, 391–416 (1941).
   P. Shubik. "Studies on the promoting phase in the stages of carcinogenesis in mice, rats, rabbits and guinea-pigs." *Cancer Res.* **10**, 13–17 (1950).

6. W. H. Hall. "The role of initiating and promoting factors in the pathogenesis of tumours of the thyroid." *Brit. J. Cancer* **2**, 273–280 (1948).

7. J. Furth and H. Sobel. "Neoplastic transformation of granulosa cells in grafts of normal ovaries into spleens of gonadectomized mice." *J. Natn. Cancer Inst.* **8**, 7–16 (1947).

8. J. K. Gong. "Anemic stress as a trigger of myelogenous leukemia in rats rendered leukemia-prone by X-ray." *Science* **174**, 833–835 (1971).

9. S. Kauffman. "Control circuits for determination and transdetermination: interpreting positional information in a binary epigenetic code." In R. Porter and J. Rivers, eds., *Cell Patterning*. Ciba Foundation Symposium 29. Elsevier, Amsterdam (1975).

10. R. K. Boutwell and D. K. Bosch. "The carcinogenicity of creosote oil: its role in the induction of skin tumors in mice." *Cancer Res.* **18**, 1171–1175 (1958).

11. K. Shanmugaratnam. "Primary carcinomas of the liver and biliary tract." *Brit. J. Cancer* **10**, 232–246 (1956).

12. J. Furth and H. Sobel. *J. Natn. Cancer Inst.* **8** (1947).

13. L. C. Stevens. "The development of transplantable teratocarcinomas from intratesticular grafts of pre- and postimplantation mouse embryos." *Devl. Biol.* **21**, 364–382 (1970).

14. B. Mintz and K. Illmensee. "Normal genetically mosaic mice produced from malignant teratocarcinoma cells." *Proc. Natn. Acad. Sci. U.S.A.* **72**, 3585–3589 (1975).
    V. E. Papaioannou, M. W. McBurney, R. L. Gardner and M. J. Evans. "Fate of teratocarcinoma cells injected into early mouse embryos." *Nature*, **258**, 70–73 (1975).

15. F. Bischoff and G. Bryson. "Carcinogenesis through solid state surfaces." *Progr. Exp. Tumor Res.* **5**, 85–133 (1964).

16. R. D. Karp et al. "Tumorigenesis by Millipore filters in mice: histology and ultrastructure of tissue reactions as related to pore size." *J. Natn. Cancer Inst.* **51**, 1275–1279 (1973).

17. L. J. Dunham. "Cancer in man at a site of prior benign lesion of skin or mucous membrane: a review." *Cancer Res.* **32**, 1359–1374 (1972).

18. H. J. Muller. "Artificial transmutation of the gene." *Science* **66**, 84–87 (1927).

19. C. Auerbach and J. M. Robson. "Chemical production of mutations." *Nature* **157**, 302 (1946).

20. S. S. Epstein. "Environmental determinants of human cancer." *Cancer Res.* **34**, 2425–2435 (1974).

21. M. Enomoto and M. Saito. "Carcinogens produced by fungi." *Ann. Rev. Microbiol.* **26**, 279–312 (1972).

22. E. Boyland. "Chemical carcinogenesis and experimental chemotherapy of cancer." *Yale J. Biol. Med.* **20**, 321–341 (1947).

23. R. E. Kouri, H. Ratrie and C. E. Whitmire. "Evidence of a genetic relationship between susceptibility to 3-methylcholanthrene-induced subcutaneous tumors and inducibility of aryl hydrocarbon hydroxylase." *J. Natn. Cancer Inst.* **51**, 197–200 (1973).

24. A. H. Conney. "Pharmacological implications of microsomal enzyme induction." *Pharmac. Rev.* **19**, 317–366 (1967).

25. E. C. Miller, J. A. Miller, R. R. Brown, and J. C. MacDonald. "On the protective action of certain polycyclic aromatic hydrocarbons against carcinogenesis by aminoazo dyes and 2-acetylaminofluorene." *Cancer Res.* **18**; 469–477 (1958).
T. L. Dao. "Inhibition of tumor induction in chemical carcinogenesis in the mammary gland." *Progr. Exp. Tumor Res.* **14**, 59–88 (1971).
D. N. Wheatley. "Enhancement and inhibition of the induction by 7,12-dimethylbenz(a)anthracene of mammary tumours in female Sprague-Dawley rats." *Brit. J. Cancer* **22**, 787–797 (1968).

26. D. W. Nebert, J. Winker, and H. V. Gelboin. "Aryl hydrocarbon hydroxylase activity in human placenta from cigarette smoking and nonsmoking women." *Cancer Res.* **29**, 1763–1769 (1969).

27. G. Kellermann, C. R. Shaw, and M. Luyten-Kellermann. Aryl-hydrocarbon-hydroxylase inducibility and bronchogenic carcinoma. *New Engl. J. Med.* **289**, 971–973 (1973).
A. E. H. Emery, et al. Aryl-hydrocarbon-hydroxylase inducibility in patients with cancer. *Lancet* **i**, 470–472 (1978).

28. A. G. Schwartz. "Correlation between species life span and capacity to activate 7,12-dimethylbenz(a)anthracene to a form mutagenic to a mammalian cell." *Exp. Cell Res.* **94**, 445–447 (1975).

29. F. Mukai and W. Troll. "The mutagenicity and initiating activity of some aromatic amine metabolites." *Ann. N.Y. Acad. Sci.* **163**, 828–836 (1969).

30. M. G. Garridge and M. S. Legator. "A host-mediated microbial assay for the detection of mutagenic compounds." *Proc. Soc. Exp. Biol. Med.* **130**, 831–834 (1969).
M. G. Garridge, A. Denunzio and M. S. Legator. "Cycasin: detection of associated mutagenic activity *in vivo.*" *Science* **163**, 689–691 (1969).

31. J. McCann, E. Choi, E. Yamasaki, and B. N. Ames. "Detection of carcinogens as mutagens in the Salmonella/microsome test: assay of 300 chemicals." *Proc. Natn. Acad. Sci. U.S.A.* **72**, 5135–5139 (1975).

32. A. Hollaender, ed. *Radiation Biology.* McGraw-Hill, New York (1954).

33. E. M. Witkin. "Ultraviolet mutagenesis and inducible DNA repair in *Escherichia coli.*" *Bact. Rev.* **40**, 869–907 (1976).

34. H. H. Rossi and A. M. Kellerer. "The validity of risk estimates of leukemia incidence based on Japanese data." *Radiat. Res.* **58**, 131–140 (1974).

35. R. Doll. *Prevention of Cancer: Pointers from Epidemiology.* The Nuffield Provincial Hospitals Trust, London (1967).

36. H. S. Kaplan, W. H. Carnes, M. B. Brown, and B. B. Hirsch. "Indirect induction of lymphomas in irradiated mice. (1) Tumor incidence and morphology in mice bearing nonirradiated thymic grafts." *Cancer Res.* **16**, 422–425 (1956).
H. S. Kaplan, B. B. Hirsch, and M. B. Brown. "Indirect induction of lymphomas in irradiated mice. (4) Genetic evidence of the origin of the tumor cells from the thymic grafts." *Cancer Res.* **16**, 434–436 (1956).
L. W. Law and M. Potter. "Further evidence of indirect induction by X-radiation of lymphocytic neoplasms in mice." *J. Natn. Cancer Inst.* **20**, 489–493 (1958).

37. J. B. Storer. Radiation carcinogenesis. In F. F. Becker, ed., *Cancer, A Comprehensive Treatise,* Volume I. Plenum Press, New York (1975).

38. F. M. Burnet. *Virus as Organism.* Harvard University Press, Cambridge, Mass. (1946).
F. Fenner et al. *The Biology of the Animal Viruses.* Academic Press, New York (1974).

39. F. L. Black. "Measles endemicity in insular populations: critical community size and its evolutionary implication." *J. Theoret. Biol.* **11**, 207–211 (1966).

40. F. Lehmann-Grube. "Lymphocytic choriomeningitis virus." *Virol. Monogr.* **10** (1971).

41. G. A. Cole, D. H. Gilden, A. A. Monjan, and N. Nathanson. "Lymphocytic choriomeningitis virus: pathogenesis of acute central nervous system disease." *Fed. Proc.* **30**, 1831–1841 (1971).

42. P. Bentvelzen. "Host-virus interactions in murine mammary carcinogenesis." *Biochim. Biophys. Acta* **355**, 236–259 (1974).

S. Nandi and C. M. McGrath. "Mammary neoplasia in mice." *Adv. Cancer Res.* **17,** 353–414 (1973).

43. L. Gross. *Oncogenic Viruses.* Pergamon Press, Oxford (1970).

44. O. Jarrett. "Evidence for the viral etiology of leukemia in the domestic mammals." *Adv. Cancer Res.* **13,** 39–62 (1970).
W. Jarrett, et al. "Antibody response and virus survival in cats vaccinated against feline leukemia." *Nature* **248,** 230–232 (1974).
M. Essex et al. "Horizontal transmission of feline leukemia virus under natural conditions in a feline leukemia cluster household." *Int. J. Cancer.* **19,** 90–96 (1977).

45. H. S. Kaplan. "On the natural history of the murine leukemias." *Cancer Res.* **27,** 1325–1340 (1967).

46. J. A. Saxton, M. C. Boon and J. Furth. "Observations on the inhibition of development of spontaneous leukemia in mice by underfeeding." *Cancer Res.* **4,** 401–409 (1944).

47. J. White and H. B. Andervont. "Effect of a diet relatively low in cystine on the production of spontaneous mammary-gland tumors in C3H female mice." *J. Natn. Cancer Inst.* **3,** 449–451 (1943).

48. W. E. Heston. Testing for possible effects of cedar wood shavings and diet on occurrence of mammary gland tumors and hepatomas in C3H-A^{vy} and C3H-A^{vy} fB mice. *J. Natn. Cancer Inst.* **54,** 1011–1014 (1975).

49. M. B. Gardner et al. "Unusually high incidence of spontaneous lymphomas in wild house mice." *J. Natn. Cancer Inst.* **50,** 1571–1579 (1973).

50. P. Bentvelzen. *Biochim. Biophys. Acta* **355,** 236–359 (1974).
S. Nandi and C. M. McGrath. *Adv. Cancer Res.* **17,** 353–414 (1973).

51. R. L. Noble and J. H. Cutts. "Mammary tumors of the rat: A review." *Cancer Res.* **19,** 1125–1139 (1959).

52. H. W. Horne. "The 'milk factor' in carcinoma of the human breast." *New Engl. J. Med.* **243,** 373–375 (1950).
J. Fraumeni and R. W. Miller. "Breast cancer and breast feeding." *Lancet* **ii,** 1196–1197 (1971)

53. H. zur Hausen. "Biochemical approaches to detection of Epstein-Barr virus in human tumors." *Cancer Res* **36,** 678–680 (1976).

54. E. Adam et al. "Seroepidemiologic studies of herpesvirus type 2 and carcinoma of the cervix. 2. Uganda." *J. Natn. Cancer Inst.* **48,** 65–72 (1972).

55. L. Aurelian, B. Schumann, R. L. Marcus, and H. J. Davis. "Antibody to HSV-2 induced tumor specific antigens in serums from patients with cervical carcinoma." *Science* **181,** 161–164 (1973).

56. D. Baltimore. "Viruses, polymerases and cancer." *Science,* **192,** 632–636 (1976).

H. M. Temin. "The DNA provirus hypothesis." *Science* **192**, 1075–1080 (1976).

57. H. M. Temin. "The protovirus hypothesis: speculations on the significance of RNA-directed DNA synthesis for normal development and for carcinogenesis." *J. Natn. Cancer Inst.* **46** iii–viii (1971)
H. M. Temin. "On the origin of RNA tumor viruses." *Ann. Rev. Genet.* **8**, 155–177 (1974).

CHAPTER 8

1. J. B. Gurdon, R. A. Laskey, and O. R. Reeves. "The developmental capacity of nuclei transplanted from keratinized skin cells of adult frogs." *J. Embryol. Exp. Morph.* **34**, 93–112 (1975).

2. G. G. Steel. "The cell cycle in tumours: an examination of data gained by the technique of labelled mitoses." *Cell and Tiss. Kinet.* **5**, 87–100 (1972).

3. O. H. Iversen, R. Bjerknes and F. Devik. "Kinetics of cell renewal, cell migration and cell loss in the hairless mouse dorsal epidermis." *Cell and Tiss. Kinet.* **1**, 351–367 (1968).
C. S. Potten. "The epidermal proliferative unit: the possible role of the central basal cell." *Cell and Tissue Kinet.* **7**, 77–88 (1974).

4. H. Quastler and F. G. Sherman. "Cell population kinetics in the intestinal epithelium of the mouse." *Exp. Cell Res.* **17**, 420–438 (1959).

5. H. Teir, T. Rytomaa, A. Cederberg, and K. Kiviniemi. "Studies on the elimination of granulocytes in the intestinal tract in rat." *Acta Path. Microbiol. Scand.* **59**, 311–324 (1963).

6. Y. Kanno and Y. Matsui. "Cellular uncoupling in cancerous stomach epithelium." *Nature* **218**, 775–776 (1968).
A. Martinez-Palomo, C. Braislovsky and W. Bernhard. Ultrastructural modifications of the cell surface and intercellular contacts of some transformed cell strains." *Cancer Res.* **29**, 925–937 (1969).
R. Azarnia and W. R. Loewenstein. "Intercellular communication and tissue growth. 5. A cancer cell strain that fails to make permeable membrane junctions with normal cells." *J. Membrane Biol.* **6**, 368–385 (1971).
R. S. Weinstein, F. B. Merk, and J. Alroy. "The structure and function of intercellular junctions in cancer." *Adv. Cancer Res.* **23**, 23–89 (1976).

7. J. C. Unkeless et al. "An enzymatic function associated with transformation of fibroblasts by oncogenic viruses. (1) Chick embryo fibroblast cultures transformed by avian RNA tumor viruses." *J. Exp. Med.* **137**, 85–111 (1973).

A. L. Latner, E. Longstaff, and K. Pradhan. "Inhibition of malignant cell invasion *in vitro* by a proteinase inhibitor." *Brit. J. Cancer* **27**, 460–464 (1973).

8. J. Folkman. "Tumor angiogenesis." *Adv. Cancer Res.* **19**, 331–358 (1974).

9. T. Gibson and W. Norris. "Skin fragments removed by injection needles." *Lancet* **ii**, 983–985 (1958).

10. N. Taptiklis. "Dormancy by dissociated thyroid cells in the lungs of mice." *Eur. J. Cancer* **4**, 59–66 (1968).

11. H. S. Micklem, C. E. Ford, E. P. Evans, and D. A. Ogden. "Compartments and cell flows within the mouse haemopoietic system. (1) Restricted interchange between haemopoietic sites." *Cell and Tiss. Kinet.* **8**, 219–232 (1975).

12. R. E. Billingham and W. K. Silvers. "Studies on the conservation of epidermal specificities of skin and certain mucosas in adult mammals." *J. Exp. Med.* **125**, 429–446 (1967).

13. R. A. Willis. *The Spread of Tumors in the Human Body.* Butterworths, London (1973).

14. L. M. Franks and T. W. Cooper. "The origin of human embryo lung cells in culture: a comment on cell differentiation, *in vitro* growth and neoplasia." *Int. J. Cancer* **9**, 19–29 (1972).
    K. R. Porter, G. J. Todaro, and V. Fonte. "A scanning electron microscope study of surface features of viral and spontaneous transformants of mouse Balb/3T3 cells." *J. Cell Biol.* **59**, 633–642 (1973).

15. L. Hayflick. "The limited *in vitro* lifetime of human diploid cell strains." *Exp. Cell Res.* **37**, 614–636 (1965).

16. P. L. Krohn. "Review lecture on senescence. (2) Heterochronic transplantation in the study of ageing." *Proc. R. Soc. Lond.* **157**, 128–147 (1962).
    L. J. T. Young, D. Medina, K. B. DeOme and C. W. Daniel. "The influence of host and tissue age on life span and growth rate of serially transplanted mouse mammary gland." *Exp. Geront.* **6**, 49–56 (1971).
    M. Rosendaal, G. S. Hodgson and T. R. Bradley. "Haemopoietic stem cells are organised for use on the basis of their generation-age." *Nature* **264**, 68–69 (1976).

17. J. G. Rheinwald and H. Green. "Epidermal growth factor and the multiplication of cultured epidermal keratinocytes." *Nature*, **265**, 421–424 (1977).

18. K. K. Sanford. "'Spontaneous' neoplastic transformation of cells *in vitro:* some facts and theories." *Natn. Cancer Inst. Monogr.* **26**, 387–418 (1967).
    R. Pollack. *Readings in Mammalian Cell Culture.* Cold Spring Harbor Laboratory, New York (1973).

19. V. Defendi, J. Lehman and P. Kraemer. "'Morphologically normal' hamster cells with malignant properties." *Virology*, **19**, 592–598 (1963).
C. W. Boone. "Malignant hemangioendotheliomas produced by subcutaneous inoculation of Balb/3T3 cells attached to glass beads." *Science* **188**, 68–70 (1975).

20. H. J. Igel, A. E. Freeman, J. E. Spiewak and K. L. Kleinfeld. "Carcinogenesis *in vitro*. (2) Chemical transformation of diploid human cell cultures: a rare event." *In Vitro* **11**, 117–129 (1975).
J. Pontén. "The relationship between *in vitro* transformation and tumor formation *in vivo*." *Biochim. Biophys. Acta* **458**, 397–422 (1976).

21. J. Thacker and R. Cox. "Mutation induction and inactivation in mammalian cells exposed to ionising radiation." *Nature* **258**, 429–431 (1975).
D. A. Spandidos and L. Siminovitch. "The relationship between transformation and somatic mutation in human and Chinese hamster cells." *Cell* **13**, 651–662 (1978).

22. Y. Berwald and L. Sachs. "*In vitro* transformation of normal cells to tumor cells by carcinogenic hydrocarbons." *J. Natn. Cancer Inst.* **35**, 641–662 (1965).

23. S. Mondal and C. Heidelberger. "Transformation of C3H/10T1/2CL8 mouse embryo fibroblasts by ultraviolet irradiation and a phorbol ester." *Nature* **260**, 710–711 (1976).

24. C. Borek and L. Sachs. "*In vitro* cell transformation by X-irradiation." *Nature* **210**, 276–278 (1966).

25. F. Fenner et al. *The Biology of the Animal Viruses*. Academic Press, New York (1974).

26. J. Tooze, ed. *The Molecular Biology of Tumour Viruses*. Cold Spring Harbor Laboratory, New York (1973).

27. P. Nevers and H. Saedler. "Transposable genetic elements as agents of gene instability and chromosomal rearrangements." *Nature* **268**, 109–115 (1977).
J. Zieg, M. Silverman, H. Hilmen, and M. Simon. "Recombinational switch for gene expression." *Science* **196**, 170–172 (1977).

28. M. Botchan, W. Topp and J. Sambrook. "The arrangement of simian virus 40 sequences in the DNA of transformed cells." *Cell* **9**, 269–287 (1976).
G. Ketner and T. J. Kelly. "Integrated simian virus 40 sequences in transformed cell DNA: analysis using restriction endonucleases." *Proc. Natn. Acad. Sci. U.S.A.* **73**, 1102–1106 (1976).

29. R. A. Weinberg. "How does T antigen transform cells?" *Cell* **11**, 243–246 (1977).

30. I. Macpherson. "The characteristics of animal cells transformed *in vitro*." *Adv. Cancer Res.* **13**, 169–215 (1970).

31. J. Pontén. "Homologous transfer of Rous sarcoma by cells." *J. Natn. Cancer Inst.* **29**, 1147–1160 (1962).

32. D. Stehelin, H. E. Varmus, J. M. Bishop, and P. K. Vogt. "DNA related to the transforming gene(s) of avian sarcoma viruses is present in normal avian DNA." *Nature* **260**, 170–173 (1976).
    T. G. Padgett, E. Stubblefield, and H. E. Varmus. "Chicken macrochromosomes contain an endogenous provirus and microchromosomes contain sequences related to the transforming gene of ASV." *Cell* **10**, 649–657 (1977).

33. R. W. Holley and J. A. Kiernan. "'Contact inhibition' of cell division in 3T3 cells." *Proc. Natn. Acad. Sci. U.S.A.* **60**, 300–304 (1968).
    R. W. Holley. "Control of growth of mammalian cells in cell culture." *Nature* **258**, 487–490 (1975).

34. G. M. Tomkins. "The metabolic code." *Science* **189**, 760–763 (1975).

35. R. O. Hynes. "Role of surface alterations in cell transformation: the importance of proteases and surface proteins." *Cell* **1**, 147–156 (1974).
    A. M. C. Rapin and M. M. Burger. "Tumor cell surfaces: general alterations detected by agglutinins." *Adv. Cancer Res.* **20**, 1–91 (1974).

36. R. Pollack, M. Osborn and K. Weber. "Patterns of organization of actin and myosin in normal and transformed cultured cells." *Proc. Natn. Acad. Sci. U.S.A.* **72**, 994–998 (1975).

37. I. Macpherson and L. Montagnier. "Agar suspension culture for the selective assay of cells transformed by polyoma virus." *Virology*, **23**, 291–294 (1964).
    S. Shin, V. H. Freedman, R. Risser, and R. Pollack. "Tumorigenicity of virus-transformed cells in *nude* mice is correlated specifically with anchorage independent growth *in vitro*." *Proc. Natn. Acad. Sci. U.S.A.* **72**, 4435–4439 (1975).

38. C. W. Boone. "Malignant hemangioendotheliomas produced by subcutaneous inoculation of Balb/3T3 cells attached to glass beads." *Science*. **188**, 68–70 (1975).

39. S. Sorieul and B. Ephrussi. "Karyological demonstration of hybridization of mammalian cells *in vitro*." *Nature* **190**, 653–654 (1961).

40. D. A. Spandidos and L. Siminovitch. "Transfer of anchorage independence by isolated metaphase chromosomes in hamster cells." *Cell* **12**, 675–682 (1977).

41. F. Wiener, G. Klein, and H. Harris. "The analysis of malignancy by cell fusion. (3) Hybrids between diploid fibroblasts and other tumour cells." *J. Cell Sci.* **8**, 681–692 (1971).
    J. Jonasson and H. Harris. "The analysis of malignancy by cell fusion. (8) Evidence for the intervention of an extra-chromosomal element." *J. Cell Sci.* **24**, 255–263 (1977).

42. J. Mark. "Chromosomal abnormalities and their specificity in human neoplasms: an assessment of recent observations by banding techniques." *Adv. Cancer Res.* **24**, 165–222 (1977).

43. P. C. Nowell and D. A. Hungerford. "Chromosome studies in human leukemia. 2. Chronic granulocytic leukemia." *J. Natn. Cancer Inst.* **27**, 1013–1036 (1961).

44. J. D. Rowley and D. Potter. "Chromosomal banding patterns in acute nonlymphocytic leukemia." *Blood* **47**, 705–721 (1976).

45. Q. V. J. Cruciger, S. Pathak and R. Cailleau. "Human breast carcinomas: marker chromosomes involving lq in seven cases." *Cytogenet. Cell Genet.* **17**, 231–235 (1976).

46. G. Manolov and Y. Manolova. "A marker band in one chromosome No. 14 in Burkitt lymphomas." *Hereditas* **69**, 300 (1971).
    L. Zech, U. Haglund, K. Nilsson, and G. Klein. "Characteristic chromosomal abnormalities in biopsies and lymphoid-cell lines from patients with Burkitt and non-Burkitt lymphomas." *Int. J. Cancer* **17**, 47–56 (1976).

47. F. M. Burnet. Self and Not-self. Cambridge University Press, London (1969).

48. "I am convinced that during development and growth malignant cells arise extremely frequently but that in the majority of people they remain latent due to the protective action of the host. I am also convinced that this natural immunity is not due to the presence of antimicrobial bodies but is determined purely by cellular factors. These may be weakened in the older age groups in which cancer is more prevalent." Paul Ehrlich (1909) (translated by Peter Alexander). From S. Himmelweit, ed., *The Collected Papers of Paul Ehrlich*, Volume 2, page 561. Pergammon Press, Oxford (1957).

49. H. O. Sjögren. "Transplantation methods as a tool for detection of tumor-specific antigens." *Progr. Exp. Tumor Res.* **6**, 289–322 (1965).
    G. Pasternak. "Antigens induced by the mouse leukemia viruses." *Adv. Cancer Res.* **12**, 1–99 (1969).

50. L. W. Law. "Immunologic responsiveness and the induction of experimental neoplasms." *Cancer Res.* **26**, 1121–1132 (1966).
    A. C. Allison and R. B. Taylor. "Observations on thymectomy and carcinogenesis." *Cancer Res.* **27**, 703–707 (1967).
    L. W. Law and S. S. Chang. "Effects of antilymphocytic serum (ALS) on the induction of lymphocytic leukemia in mice." *Proc. Soc. Exp. Biol. Med.* **136**, 420–425 (1971).

51. M. Essex et al. "Horizontal transmission of feline leukemia virus under natural conditions in a feline leukemia cluster household." *Int. J. Cancer* **19**, 90–96 (1977).

52. G. Klein, H. O. Sjögren, E. Klein and K. E. Hellström. "Demonstra-

tion of resistance against methylcholanthrene-induced sarcomas in the primary autochthonous host." *Cancer Res.* **20**, 1561–1572 (1960).

53. R. T. Prehn and J. M. Main. "Immunity to methylcholanthrene-induced sarcomas." *J. Natn. Cancer Inst.* **18**, 769–778 (1957).
R. T. Prehn. "Relationship of tumor immunogenicity to concentration of the oncogen." *J. Natn. Cancer Inst.* **55**, 189–190 (1975).

54. J. L. Wagner and G. Haughton. "Immunosuppression by anti-lymphocyte serum and its effect on tumors induced by 3-methylcholanthrene in mice." *J. Natn. Cancer Inst.* **46**, 1–10 (1971).
O. Stutman. "Tumor development after 3-methylcholanthrene in immunologically deficient athymic-nude mice." *Science* **183**, 534–536 (1974).

55. I. Penn and T. E. Starzl. "A summary of the status of *de novo* cancer in transplant recipients." *Transplant. Proc.* **4**, 719–732 (1972).
R. Hoover and J. F. Fraumeni. "Risk of cancer in renal-transplant recipients." *Lancet* **ii**, 55–57 (1973).
A. J. Matas, R. L. Simmons and J. S. Najarian. "Chronic antigenic stimulation, herpesvirus infection, and cancer in transplant recipients." *Lancet* **i**, 1277–1279 (1975).

56. J. H. Kersey, B. D. Spector and R. A. Good. "Primary immunodeficiency diseases and cancer: the immunodeficiency-cancer registry." *Int. J. Cancer* **12**, 333–347 (1973).

57. I. C. Roberts-Thompson, S. Whittingham, U. Youngchaiyud, and I. R. Mackay. "Ageing, immune response, and mortality." *Lancet* **ii**, 368–370 (1974).

58. S. Shapiro, O. P. Heinonen, and V. Siskind. "Cancer and allergy." *Cancer* **28**, 396–400 (1971).
A. P. Polednak. "Asthma and cancer mortality." *Lancet* **ii**, 1147–1148 (1975).

59. E. R. Pund and S. H. Auerbach. "Pre-invasive carcinoma of the cervix uteri." *J. Am. Med. Assn.* **131**, 960–963 (1946).
Z. W. Zagula-Mally, E. W. Rosenberg, and M. Kashgarian. "Frequency of skin cancer and solar keratoses in a rural southern county as determined by population sampling." *Cancer* **34**, 345–349 (1974).

60. R. Doll and L. Kinlen. "Immunosurveillance and cancer: epidemiological evidence." *Brit. Med. J.* **iv**, 420–422 (1970).

61. E. S. Spencer and H. K. Andersen. "Clinically evident, non-terminal infections with herpesviruses and the wart virus in immunosuppressed renal allograft recipients." *Brit. Med. J.* **iii**, 251–254 (1970).

62. J. H. Coggin and N. G. Anderson. "Cancer, differentiation and embryonic antigens: some central problems." *Adv. Cancer Res.* **19**, 105–165 (1974).

63. D. P. Stevens. I. R. Mackay, and K. J. Cullen. "Carcinoembryonic antigen in an unselected elderly population: a four year follow up." *Brit. J. Cancer* **32**, 147–151 (1975).
R. R. Williams et al. "Tumor-associated antigen levels (carcinoembryonic antigen, human chorionic gonadotropin, and alpha-fetoprotein) antedating the diagnosis of cancer in the Framingham study." *J. Natn. Cancer Inst.* **58**, 1547–1551 (1977).

CHAPTER 9

1. W. M. Court Brown and R. Doll. "Mortality from cancer and other causes after radiotherapy for ankylosing spondylitis." *Brit. Med. J.* **ii**, 1327–1332 (1965).
I. Mackenzie. "Breast cancer following multiple fluoroscopies." *Brit. J. Cancer* **19**, 1–8 (1965).

2. A. L. Herbst, H. Ulfelder and D. C. Poskanzer. "Adenocarcinoma of the vagina. Association of maternal stilbestrol therapy with tumor appearance in young women." *New Engl. J. Med.* **284**, 878–881 (1971).

3. P. Armitage and R. Doll. "The age distribution of cancer and a multi-stage theory of carcinogenesis." *Brit. J. Cancer* **8**, 1–12 (1954).

4. A. C. Allison, F. C. Chesterman and S. Baron. "Induction of tumors in adult hamsters with simian virus 40." *J. Natn. Cancer Inst.* **38**, 567–572 (1967).

5. B. MacMahon, P. Cole, and J. Brown. "Etiology of human breast cancer: a review." *J. Natn. Cancer Inst.* **50**, 21–42 (1973).

6. I. J. Selikoff, E. C. Hammond, and J. Churg. "Asbestos exposure, smoking, and neoplasia." *J. Amer. Med. Assn.* **204**, 106–112 (1968).
G. Berry, M. L. Newhouse, and M. Turok. "Combined effect of asbestos exposure and smoking on mortality from lung cancer in factory workers." *Lancet* **ii**, 476–479 (1972).

7. F. A. Langley and A. C. Crompton. "Epithelial abnormalities of the cervix uteri." *Recent Results in Cancer Research,* Vol. 40 (1973).

8. R. M. Richart. "Colpomicroscopic studies of cervical intraepithelial neoplasia." *Cancer* **19**, 395–405 (1966).

9. L. G. Koss et al. "Some histological aspects of behavior of epidermoid carcinoma in situ and related lesions of the uterine cervix." *Cancer* **16**, 1160–1211 (1963).

10. R. M. Richart. "A radioautographic analysis of cellular proliferation in dysplasia and carcinoma in situ of the uterine cervix." *Amer. J. Obstet. Gynec.* **86**, 925–930 (1963).
H. F. Schellhas. "Cell renewal in the human cervix uteri." *Amer. J. Obstet. Gynec.* **104**, 617–632 (1969).

11. J. E. Dunn. "The presymptomatic diagnosis of cancer with special reference to cervical cancer." *Proc. R. Soc. Med.* **59**, 1198–1204 (1966).
B. A. Barron and R. M. Richart. "A statistical model of the natural history of cervical carcinoma based on a prospective study of 557 cases." *J. Natn. Cancer Inst.* **41**, 1343–1353 (1968).
B. A. Barron and R. M. Richart. "A statistical model of the natural history of cervical carcinoma. (2) Estimates of the transition time from dysplasia to carcinoma in situ." *J. Natn. Cancer Inst.* **45**, 1025–1030 (1970).

12. O. Petersen. "Spontaneous course of cervical precancerous conditions." *Amer. J. Obstet. Gynec.* **72**, 1063–1071 (1956).
A. I. Spriggs. "Follow-up of untreated carcinoma-in-situ of cervix uteri." *Lancet* **ii**, 599–600 (1971).

13. T. C. Everson. "Spontaneous regression of cancer." *Ann. N.Y. Acad. Sci.* **114**, 721–735 (1964).

14. R. Bangle, M. Berger and M. Levin. "Variations in the morphogenesis of squamous carcinoma of the cervix." *Cancer* **16**, 1151–1159 (1963).

15. B. Halpert, E. E. Sheehan, W. R. Schmalhorst, and R. Scott. "Carcinoma of the prostate. A survey of 5000 autopsies." *Cancer* **16**, 737–742 (1963).

16. Z. W. Zagula-Mally, E. W. Rosenberg, and M. Kashgarian. "Frequency of skin cancer and solar keratoses in a rural southern county as determined by population sampling." *Cancer* **34**, 345–349 (1974).

17. I. Park and H. W. Jones. "Glucose-6-phosphate dehydrogenase and the histogenesis of epidermoid carcinoma of the cervix." *Amer. J. Obstet. Gynec.* **102**, 106–109 (1968).

18. J. E. Enstrom and D. F. Austin. "Interpreting cancer survival rates." *Science* **195**, 847–851 (1977).

19. *Vital Statistics of the United States.* U.S. Dept. of Health, Education, and Welfare, Washington, D.C.

20. S. J. Cutler, M. H. Myers, and S. B. Green. "Trends in survival rates of patients with cancer." *New Engl. J. Med.* **293**, 122–124 (1975).

21. J. E. Enstrom and D. F. Austin. *Science* **195**, 847–851 (1977).

22. L. Venet, P. Strax, W. Venet and S. Shapiro. "Adequacies and inadequacies of breast examinations by physicians in mass screening." *Cancer* **28**, 1546–1551 (1971).

23. P. Strax. "Control of breast cancer through mass screening." *J. Amer. Med. Assn.* **235**, 1600–1602 (1976).

24. A. M. Lilienfeld, M. L. Levin, and I. I. Kessler. *Cancer in the United States.* Harvard University Press. Cambridge, Mass. (1972).

25. C. E. Marshall. "A ten-year cervical-smear screening programme." *Lancet* **ii**, 1026–1029 (1968).

A. B. Miller, J. Lindsay, and G. B. Hill. "Mortality from cancer of the uterus in Canada and its relationship to screening for cancer of the cervix." *Int. J. Cancer* **17**, 602–612 (1976).

CHAPTER 10

1. A. B. Miller, J. Lindsay, and G. B. Hill. "Mortality from cancer of the uterus in Canada and its relationship to screening for cancer of the cervix." *Int. J. Cancer* **17**, 602–612 (1976).

2. G. Z. Brett. "Earlier diagnosis and survival in lung cancer." *Brit. Med. J.* **iv**, 260–262 (1969).

3. P. Strax. "Control of breast cancer through mass screening." *J. Amer. Med. Assn.* **235**, 1600–1602 (1976).

4. T. A. Hodgson. "The economic costs of cancer." In D. Schottenfeld, ed. *Cancer Epidemiology and Prevention: Current Concepts.* C. C. Thomas, Springfield, Illinois (1975).

5. L. Howard, C. C. Erickson, and L. D. Stoddard. "A study of the incidence and histogenesis of endocervical metaplasia and intra-epithelial carcinoma." *Cancer* **4**, 1210–1223 (1951).
   J. D. Mortensen, W. A. Bennett, and L. B. Woolner. "Incidence of carcinoma in thyroid glands removed at 1000 consecutive routine necropsies." *Sci. Forum* **5**, 659–663 (1954).
   L. M. Franks. "Latency and progression in tumours: the natural history of prostatic cancer." *Lancet* **ii**, 1037–1039 (1956).
   A. J. M. Reese and D. P. Winstanley. "The small tumour-like lesions of the kidney." *Brit. J. Cancer* **12**, 507–516 (1958).
   B. Halpert, E. E. Sheehan, W. R. Schmalhorst, and R. Scott. "Carcinoma of the prostate. A survey of 5000 autopsies." *Cancer* **16**, 737–742 (1963).
   T. C. Arminski and D. W. McLean. "Incidence and distribution of adenomatous polyps of the colon and rectum based on 1000 autopsy examinations." *Dis. Colon Rectum* **7**, 249–261 (1964).

6. A. G. Knudson. "Mutation and human cancer." *Adv. Cancer Res.* **17**, 317–352 (1973).

7. J. F. Fraumeni, ed. *Persons at High Risk of Cancer.* Academic Press, London (1975).

8. M. J. Hill et al. "Faecal bile acids and Clostridia in patients with cancer of the large bowel." *Lancet* **i**, 535–539 (1975).

9. R. R. Williams et al. "Tumor-associated antigen levels (carcino-embryonic antigen, human chorionic gonadotropin, and alpha-feto-protein) antedating the diagnosis of cancer in the Framingham study." *J. Natn. Cancer Inst.* **58**, 1547–1551 (1977).

10. K. D. Bagshawe. "Recent observations related to the chemotherapy and immunology of gestational choriocarcinoma." *Adv. Cancer Res.* **18,** 231–263 (1973).

11. M. Lalonde. *A New Perspective on the Health of Canadians.* Canadian Government, Ottawa (1975).

12. R. L. Phillips. "Role of life-style and dietary habits in the risk of cancer among seventh-day adventists." *Cancer Res.* **35,** 3513–3522 (1975).

13. E. L. Wynder and D. Hoffmann. "The tenth anniversary of the Surgeon General's report on smoking and health: Have we made any progress?" *J. Natn. Cancer Inst.* **54,** 533–534 (1975).

14. Department of Health and Social Security. *Smoking and Health; a Study of the Effects of a Reduction in Cigarette Smoking on Mortality and Morbidity Rates, on Health Care and Social Security Expenditure and on Productive Potential.* H. M. Stationary Office, London (1972).

15. I. D. Bross and R. Gibson. "Risks of lung cancer in smokers who switch to filter cigarettes." *Amer. J. Publ. Hlth.* **58,** 1396–1403 (1968). E. C. Hammond, L. Garfinkel, H. Seidman and E. A. Lew. "Tar and nicotine content of cigarette smoke in relation to death rates." *Environ. Res.* **12,** 263–274 (1976).

16. E. Yamasaki and B. N. Ames. "Concentration of mutagens from urine by adsorption with the nonpolar resin XAD-2: Cigarette smokers have mutagenic urine." *Proc. Natn. Acad. Sci. U.S.A.* **74,** 3555–3559 (1977).

17. L. Thomas. "Biomedical science and human health: the long-range prospect." *Daedalus* (Summer 1977).

INDEX